Ocular Anatomy and Physiology

Second Edition

Ocular Anatomy and Physiology

Second Edition

Al Lens, COMT

Pro-lens Ophthalmic Services
Vancouver, BC

Sheila Coyne Nemeth, COMT

Eye of the Wolf, LLC
Rio Rancho, NM

Janice K. Ledford, COMT

EyeWrite Productions
Franklin, NC

Series Editors

Janice K. Ledford, COMT • Ken Daniels, OD • Robert Campbell, MD

SLACK
INCORPORATED

Delivering the best in health care information and education worldwide

www.Healio.com/books

ISBN: 978-1-55642-792-3

The previous edition of this book was published as *Ocular Anatomy and Physiology* by Al Lens, Tammy Langley, Sheila Coyne Nemeth, and Carolyn Shea.

Published by: SLACK Incorporated
6900 Grove Road
Thorofare, NJ 08086 USA
Telephone: 856-848-1000
Fax: 856-853-5991
www.slackbooks.com

Library of Congress Cataloging-in-Publication Data

Lens, Al.
Ocular anatomy and physiology / Al Lens, Sheila Coyne Nemeth, Janice K. Ledford. -- 2nd ed.
p. ; cm.
Rev. ed. of: Ocular anatomy and physiology / Al Lens ... [et al.]. c1999.
Includes bibliographical references and index.
ISBN 978-1-55642-792-3 (alk. paper)
1. Eye--Physiology. 2. Eye--Anatomy. 3. Eye-sockets. I. Nemeth, Sheila Coyne. II. Ledford, Janice K. III. Ocular anatomy and physiology. IV. Title.
[DNLM: 1. Eye--anatomy & histology--Examination Questions. 2. Diagnostic Techniques, Ophthalmological--Examination Questions. 3. Ocular Physiology--Examination Questions. 4. Vision Disorders--Examination Questions. WW 101 L573o 2007]

QP475.O28 2007
612.8'4--dc22

2007032218

Printed in the United States of America.

Last digit is print number: 10 9 8 7 6 5 4 3 2

Dedication, Second Edition

For Dr. Charles Kirby and Jane, with deep appreciation.
Jan Ledford

To my children, Natalie and Ben:
May God always hold you in the palm of His hand.
Sheila Coyne Nemeth

Dedication, First Edition

There has been one person who has demonstrated more faith in what I may have to offer to this wonderful profession than any one else. To her, I dedicate my portion of this book with love and gratitude. Thanks, Jan … more.
Tammy Langley

To my father, Phil Coyne,
whose sense of humor and adaptability to life's journey is truly heroic.
Sheila Coyne Nemeth

Contents

Acknowledgments, Second Edition

My appreciation for those whose assistance made this work possible is limitless. Thank you to the original authors of the material and to the team in the book division of SLACK Incorporated. (SLACK Incorporated has been especially patient with the delays that have plagued this second edition.)

The word *gratitude* falls far short in describing what I owe Charles Kirby, MD and Jane Kirby, RN. Not only have they supported me as a colleague in patient care, but they have given me the priceless gift of their friendship as well. Without their encouragement and understanding, putting one foot in front of the other would be nearly impossible.

Jan Ledford

In this most interesting phase of my eye career, I would like to thank many of the great souls I have worked with these past years as Eye of the Wolf has continued to evolve: Paul and Cathy Truitt for Elsa; Paul Foumier for his great spirits, great cooking, and optical brilliance; Steve Russell for energy when there was little; Desi and Pearly for walking the long pilgrimage each year to Chimayo; Gilberto for his stamina and support; Leona for her love of life; Linda Mola for her joy of the eccentric Irish humor of life; Peter and Susan Soliz for being there; Ana Edwards for her artistic translations of complex ideas; and Arup Das for his continued mentoring of the entire universe.

As always, thanks to my husband George for holding on through the continued chaos and piles of papers, and to my teenaged children, Ben and Natalie, who will always have my heart wherever the chaos takes me.

Sheila Coyne Nemeth, COMT

Acknowledgments, First Edition

It is a pleasure to acknowledge the people who have made my chapters possible. First, without the generosity of Dr. Howard Gimbel, I would not have had the opportunity to work in ophthalmology. Judy Gimbel encouraged me to write *The Ophthalmic Assisting Guide*, followed several years later with the second edition. I am indebted to my family (my wife, Sheila, and my daughters, Bridgette and Meagan), who have been supportive during all the days and nights I spent writing. And, of course, my appreciation to Jan Ledford—the editor of this wonderful series—who has been kindly critiquing my work.

Al Lens, COMT

I would like to thank Dr. Johnny Gayton for having been a faithful teacher over many years; Dr. Richard Eisner for lending his professional ear; Dr. Monte Murphy for allowing me to use his personal library for research; Todd Lowery for his example; Val Sanders for always being there to offer a new way to look at things; and especially to Jim, Josh, and Chris who give perspective to all I do.

Tammy Langley, COT

I wish to acknowledge the support of the Division of Ophthalmology at the University of New Mexico Health Sciences Center—especially our chief, Dr. Mark Schluter, who was always available to act as my editor, and who continually encourages personal academic endeavors. Drs. Greg Ogawa, Denise Farnath, Arup Das, Mark Wood, and Randi Thompson were also continuous support systems for resources and moral support. My great "tech" friends Maurice, Pearl, Rocky, Anna, Liz, Marla, and Gene always gave me cheers through days when there was no more time left to fit in this extra work. My nurse manager, Rita Sue, always was there to listen.

I wish to express my gratitude to Dr. Peter Soliz at Kestrel Corporation for helping me expand my horizons into the research arena for future ophthalmic innovations. His dauntless commitment to research is honorable.

Last, but never least, is my family, whose house is never as "kept" as it should be with a working/author wife/mother. My husband, George, has learned to close his eyes, and my great children, Ben and Natalie, have learned to be creative within the chaos. They are my best support system of all.

Sheila Coyne Nemeth, COMT

In my 20-year journey in ophthalmology, there have been many special people who have encouraged, supported, and inspired me. Unfortunately, there is not enough space to thank all of them, but you know who you are.

Specific recognition goes to my parents, who have continued to support me; Norma Garber, COMT, BA, for without her in my life I would be sad; the ophthalmology staff, MDs, techs, and support staff who have stood by me in good and bad times; the women of Shepard House who gave me my life back; and Kay, for being there for me.

Carolyn Shea, COMT

About the Authors

Al Lens, COMT, began his career in ophthalmology in 1986 at the Gimbel Eye Centre in Calgary, Alberta, Canada. He developed a comprehensive training program to teach new ophthalmic assistants at the clinic where he worked. He then began lecturing at various conferences across North America and Saudi Arabia. His other published works include *Ophthalmic Assisting Guide; Optics, Retinoscopy and Refractometry, Second Edition; LASIK for Technicians*; and *Cataract and Glaucoma for Eyecare Paraprofessionals*. Currently, Al works at various clinics in Vancouver, British Columbia, Canada.

Sheila Coyne Nemeth, COMT, received her Bachelor of Arts degree in English literature from the University of New Hampshire and graduated from the Boston University Ophthalmic Technology program. Her career path has included working with Phoenix Indian Medical Center in Phoenix, Arizona, and as a program director of ophthalmic technology at the Eastern Virginia Medical School in Norfolk, Virginia.

Currently, she resides in Corrales, New Mexico, where she has a consulting company called Eye of the Wolf LLC. She has been coauthor and researcher on multiple National Institute of Health research grants, with an interest in image processing analysis of retinal images. Her husband George and her two teenagers, Ben and Natalie, keep her quite active.

Janice K. Ledford, COMT, has become well known in ophthalmic assisting circles, especially among those studying for certification exams. Her many text books and articles continue to contribute to the field of eye care. In addition to writing, editing, and teaching, Jan works for Dr. Charles Kirby as well as the Veterans Administration Eye Clinic in Asheville, North Carolina. She lives in the mountains of North Carolina with her two cats. Next time you see her, she would love to tell you about her kids and grandkids.

Contributing Authors

R. Rand Allingham, MD
Director, Glaucoma Service
Associate Professor, Ophthalmology
Duke University Medical Center
Durham, NC

Mark DiSclafani, MD
Glaucoma Specialist
The Eye Associates
Bradenton, FL

Tammy Langley, COT
Cool Smiles
Macon, GA

Mark Schluter, MD
Associate Professor
University of New Mexico Health Sciences Center
School of Medicine
Division of Ophthalmology
Albuquerque, NM

Carolyn Shea, COMT
Manager
The Glaucoma Consultation Service
Massachusetts Eye and Ear Infirmary
Boston, MA

Introduction

The eye is one of the body's most fascinating structures. It is thrilling to observe and learn about; it may not be so thrilling to write about. The authors who wrote this book faced a special challenge. They were originally told to describe normal ocular anatomy and physiology while keeping discussion on abnormalities to a bare minimum.

This was a difficult task because often we learn as much about what is "normal" by learning about what is abnormal. They have done an admirable job. For this second edition, we have added a glossary of common disorders to appropriate chapters. For further material on ocular disorders, please see Basic Bookshelf titles *Overview of Ocular Disorder*s and *Emergencies in Eyecare*.

There have also been some changes regarding the book's authors. Both Tammy Langley and Carolyn Shea, who wrote for the first edition, elected to opt out this time around. Their portions of the text have been updated by the remaining two original authors (Al Lens and Sheila Coyne Nemeth) and Jan Ledford.

A few other notes are worthwhile here. If you are familiar with other books in *The Basic Bookshelf for Eyecare Professionals*, you will notice that the study icons are missing from this particular volume. (The study icons are symbols that appear in the margins to indicate that adjacent material is a content area on a certification examination. Examinations included are the three levels of ophthalmic assisting, the two levels of optometric assisting, plus contact lenses, opticianry, ophthalmic photography, low vision, and surgical assisting.) This deletion is due to ambiguity on the part of the test criteria; most of the exam criteria list "ocular anatomy and physiology" as a blanket phrase. Thus, for us to assign icons, we would have to second-guess the commissions and committees who put the exams together. We were not willing to do this. The best we can say is that portions of this book may be more advanced than certain examinations require. However, we have done our best to ensure that all the material that we judged may be needed for the higher-level exams is included.

Another *Basic Bookshelf* feature is the patient education sidebars. These are boxed areas of text that tell the assistant (or whomever) what to tell the patient regarding a procedure, a treatment, or a disorder. Again, this feature has not been included in this particular text. Surely most every office and clinic will have an eye model or pictures with which to explain the appropriate ocular anatomy to the patient. Obviously, when discussing anatomy with a layman, be careful to use words and language that the patient can relate to (ie, say "white of the eye" instead of "sclera").

We trust that these few changes have made this book even more useful to you, and that you will continue to consult *Basic Bookshelf* titles as you expand your knowledge about this fascinating subject.

Janice K. (Jan) Ledford, COMT
Series Editor, *The Basic Bookshelf for Eyecare Professionals*

Chapter 1

Ocular Anatomy and Physiology Jump-Start

Al Lens, COMT

It has been said that the eyes are the windows to the soul. You can tell a lot about people by watching their eyes: whether they are happy, sad, angry, or even lying. This book will not teach you any of that! What *will* be covered is the parts of the eye and their functions. This first chapter is an overview of the anatomy and physiology of the eye, and each following chapter is more in-depth.

Anatomy of the Eye

The eyes are sophisticated organs that we rely on heavily to help us process our world. Because they are so vital, the eyes are quite well protected. Each eyeball (or globe) is surrounded by a bony orbit to prevent trauma to the eye by larger objects. There are seven different bones comprising each orbit, some more fragile than others and thus more prone to fracture (see Chapter 3 for more details on the bony orbit).

The size of the eyeball or globe does not vary much after 2 years of age. The need for corrective lenses, and how strong those lenses are, often correlates to the size of the globe. When the body grows, the eyeball may also grow (elongate) and cause nearsightedness or myopia. Eyes that are smaller (shorter) than average are typically farsighted or hyperopic.

Above each eye, the eyebrow diverts sweat from the forehead away from the eye. The eyelashes detect smaller objects close to the eye; the lids close quickly when the lashes sense danger. Of course, the eyes themselves will often see a threat approaching and will close the eyelids for protection.

The eyelids also spread the tears across the eye. The lacrimal gland that produces the watery part of the tears is situated above the eye toward the outer edge, under the brow. When the lids blink, the tears are pushed across the eye toward the nose. Conveniently, there are little drain holes, called puncta, in the upper and lower lids close to the nose that carry away excess tears. This drainage system makes its way into the nose, explaining why our nose runs when we cry. (See Chapter 4 for more details on the eyebrows, eyelids, and the lacrimal system.)

It would not be very useful to have eyes that could not adjust their position. Attached to each eye are six extraocular muscles that move the eye up, down, left, right, and diagonally. They can even rotate the globe to a certain degree as the head is tipped sideways. Sometimes the innervation of the muscles (the signal from the brain) does not match up between the two eyes and they become misaligned, causing a condition called strabismus. Nobody has figured out a way to change the signal strength from the brain, so when strabismus occurs, eye muscle surgery is performed to adjust the length of the muscle(s) to compensate for the nerve problem.

Both eyes have to be looking at the same object to have good binocular depth perception. In strabismus, each eye sees a different image, creating double vision. When strabismus occurs in childhood, the brain will suppress one of the disparate images to eliminate diplopia. If the suppression continues undetected into the preteen years, the eye that has been "turned off" will have irreparable problems with vision (amblyopia). (See Chapter 5 for more information on the extraocular muscles.)

The bulbar conjunctiva is a mucous membrane that covers the sclera (the white of the eye). This membrane is continuous with the palpebral conjunctiva, which lines the eyelids, so objects (eg, contact lenses) cannot disappear behind the eye. The episclera is right under the bulbar conjunctiva and is rich with blood vessels. These vessels nourish the underlying sclera. The contents of the eye are held together mostly by the sclera, which is composed of dense collagen fibers. Any of these structures can become inflamed, and the eye can then appear red due to the dilated blood vessels. (See Chapter 6 for more information on the conjunctiva, episclera, and sclera.)

The "window" of the eye is the cornea. This structure is responsible for about two-thirds of the eye's focusing power. The area of strongest focusing power, and thinnest part of the cornea, is its center. There are five layers of the cornea and each has its own function. The only layer with any ability to regenerate its cells is the outermost layer, the epithelium. A corneal abrasion results when the epithelium detaches from Bowman's membrane (usually due to trauma); the pain can be intense, but once the epithelium restores itself, no evidence of the injury will remain. Damage to the stroma, which accounts for 90% of the corneal thickness, will result in a scar. (See Chapter 7 for more information on the cornea.)

Inside the eye are two segments—the anterior and posterior. The anterior segment is further divided into two chambers—the anterior and posterior. (The segments and chambers are sometimes confused.) The front or anterior chamber is filled with aqueous, a fluid that provides nutrition to the areas lacking blood vessels (ie, the crystalline lens and the cornea). The iris (colored part of the eye) separates the anterior chamber from the posterior chamber. The opening in the middle of the iris is known as the pupil. The size of the pupil adjusts according to the level of light and accommodation (focusing) using the iris sphincter and dilator muscles.

In the posterior chamber, the crystalline lens is suspended by very thin fibers called zonules. These are attached to the ciliary muscle, which contracts and dilates to adjust the power of the lens to vary the focus from far to near or vice-versa. Unfortunately, the lens loses the ability to change its focus with each passing year. By age 45, most people experience difficulty with near focus, while their distance vision remains clear; this is known as presbyopia. The lens continues to undergo changes and will eventually develop a cataract, which is a clouding of the normally-clear lens tissue, causing decreased vision. The ciliary body and iris (along with the choroid, discussed next) collectively make up the uvea. (See Chapter 8 for more information and the anterior and posterior chambers.)

The posterior segment is behind the anterior segment, consisting of the vitreous, posterior sclera, choroid, and retina. The jelly-like vitreous does not really seem to serve a great purpose except to fill the cavity. The choroid, which is rich with blood vessels, provides all the nourishment for the retina's photoreceptors.

The human eye has two types of photoreceptors: rods and cones. Rods function in dim lighting at night. The cone cells function in daylight conditions. The rods do not have any color perception, which is why we cannot pick out coordinating clothes in the dark. The macula, a special area of the retina, is aligned with our central line of sight and has a high concentration of cones. This allows us to see great detail centrally. (Our peripheral vision is around 20/200 or 20/400, not suitable for reading.)

About 15 degrees nasal to the macula is the optic disk (also called the optic nerve head) where the nerve fibers exit the eye and extend to the brain. The central retinal vein also exits the eye here and the central retinal artery enters here. There are no photoreceptors in the optic disk, so this is the source of our physiologic blind spot (which appears 15 degrees temporal to fixation and just a little below the horizontal midline). (See Chapter 9 for more information on the posterior segment.)

The eyeball is a receptor for information which is then sent to the brain. The "path of light" refers to light as it passes through the globe. It begins with the tear film, then travels through the cornea, aqueous, pupil, lens, vitreous, and the retina. Vision itself actually begins in the occipital cortex in the posterior aspect of the brain.

If something happens to nerve fibers anywhere between the eye and the brain, defects in the visual field will occur. (The visual field is the area of vision that is visible around the point of fixation, typically extending about 95 degrees temporally, 65 degrees nasally and superiorly, and 75 degrees inferiorly, depending on facial features that restrict peripheral vision.) Knowing how the incoming image is affected at each stage along the visual pathway helps the examiner determine where nerve damage has occurred based on visual field defects. This can be done because different parts of the visual pathway affect specific parts of the visual field. For example, brain tumors can sometimes be detected through analysis of the visual field. (See Chapter 10 for more information on the visual pathway.)

Humans have 12 pairs of cranial nerves (CN). Seven of these affect vision (CN II to VIII), some more perceptibly than others. The optic nerve (CN II) is probably the most important as it is responsible for sight. CNs III, IV, and VI are responsible for innervating the extraocular muscles. CN V provides sensation of touch in a good portion of the facial area, including the eyes. CN VII provides reflex tearing and blinking. Damage to a specific part of CN VIII can result in nystagmus (ie, rhythmic, involuntary eye movements). (See Chapter 11 for more information on cranial nerves.)

Physiology of the Eye

Vision is a complex chain of events. Light passes through the optical media of the eye (cornea, aqueous, crystalline lens, and vitreous) and stimulates the photoreceptors that send the signal to the brain through the visual pathway. The brain then recognizes the image, interprets what has been seen, and responds accordingly. However, vision does not end there; the eyes have to maintain alignment with each other (fusion) so that the part of the visual field that overlaps does not cause double vision, and we can have depth perception.

There are three degrees of fusion. The first degree occurs when the image from a single eye is superimposed over the image from the other eye. The next degree is when there is flat fusion and a two-dimensional image is formed. Third degree fusion provides binocular depth perception.

Unlike many animals, the human visual field has a considerable amount of overlap (about 120 degrees). This overlap is part of what gives humans superior depth perception. Interestingly enough, the left side of the visual field (toward the ear in the left eye and toward the nose in the right eye) is seen by the right side of the brain, and vice-versa. This occurs because the nerves from the nasal side of each eye cross over; this happens at the optic chiasm, an area of the brain that lies underneath the pituitary gland. A lesion in this area would cause a defect to the temporal side of the visual field in each eye because the nasal fibers are responsible for temporal vision. Since the nerve fibers from the retina to the brain are arranged in a specific way, a visual field defect can often indicate what part of the visual path is affected.

Accommodation is the ability of the eye to increase its focusing power for close objects. The crystalline lens becomes more round in shape (effectively adding plus power) as the ciliary muscle contracts. Accommodation also plays a role in depth perception as the brain uses the amount of focusing exerted to gauge the distance to an object. When accommodation takes place, the eyes also converge (move inward) and the pupil gets smaller. This combination of events is sometimes called the accommodative reflex, although it is not a true reflex.

Refractive Errors

While the majority of people can see clearly in the distance without having to wear glasses or contact lenses, most eyes do have at least a slight refractive error (or lack of clear focus). The most common refractive error is astigmatism, but it usually exists in such a low amount that it is not noticeable in everyday life. Astigmatism is a refractive error that is not equal in all meridians and thus causes the object of focus to be blurred. It is commonly caused by a cornea that is not spherical.

The next most common refractive error is myopia, or nearsightedness. Eyes that are myopic can see clearly at some point closer than infinity (near objects) and the distant vision is unclear.

Hyperopia, or farsightedness, is present in most humans at birth, but the eye's ability to change its focus (accommodation) at this early age brings objects into focus anyway. However, if a hyperopic eye is in a relaxed state, objects at *any* distance appear blurry: the closer the object, the more unclear it is.

Around the age of 45 most people start to notice that they cannot accommodate enough to be able to change their focus from the distance to a nearby object (computers, reading material, etc). This is known as presbyopia, which is generally corrected with reading glasses (or a bifocal, if the person is already wearing glasses).

Common Myths

There are many myths about the eyes that seem to get passed down from generation to generation. Listed below are some of the most common myths and the truths regarding them.

- Myth #1: Reading in the dark will hurt your eyes. Fact: This is no more true than taking pictures in the dark will ruin a camera. Granted, it is more difficult to see in dim light, but it will not cause any harm to your eyes.
- Myth #2: You should avoid using your eyes too much or you will wear them out. Fact: Studies have shown that this is far from the truth. In reality, it appears that those who do not use their eyes regularly for fine detail (such as reading and other close work) are more likely to develop macular degeneration, a disease that affects central vision.
- Myth #3: If you cross your eyes, they will get stuck that way. Fact: The same muscles that move the eyes to the left and right are used to converge the eyes (ie, bring them both in, toward the nose). If crossing the eyes would make them get stuck, then the same caution would have to apply to moving the eyes any direction.
- Myth #4: It will hurt a child's eyes to sit too close to the television set. Fact: A television set is quite similar to a cathode ray tube screen or computer monitor, from which adults sit an arm's length away for many hours a day! Children like to sit close to the screen to feel more involved in the show, but it will not damage their eyes.
- Myth #5: If you only have one good eye, you should avoid overworking it. Fact: One eye cannot compensate, or work harder, because the other eye is not working so well. It would be like saying that if you lose some hearing in one ear, the other ear has to work harder. Like the ear, the eye can only perform to its ability, no more, no less.
- Myth #6: You can have your eyes transplanted. Fact: Corneal transplants are common, but it is not possible to reconnect the millions of nerves that connect the eye to the brain.
- Myth #7: When surgery is performed on the eye, the eye is removed, repaired, and then reinserted. Fact: See answer to Myth #6, above.
- Myth #8: Cataracts actually improve your vision. Fact: A cloudy lens cannot technically improve vision, but many people discover that they suddenly have the ability to read without glasses! Most cataracts cause a myopic shift (the eye becomes more nearsighted). Those who previously wore reading glasses find they can read without them, but their distance vision typically becomes blurry. At some point, the cataract will become dense enough that the vision is too cloudy to be able to read with or without glasses.
- Myth #9: You have to wait for a cataract to be "ripe" before having it removed. Fact: This was true many years ago because the entire lens (including the capsular bag) was removed and it was easier if the lens was hardened by the dense cataract. Now, it is much safer to remove the cataract before it gets really dense due to the more sophisticated instruments that break the cataract into tiny pieces and suction them away.
- Myth #10: Cataracts can be removed with a laser. Fact: Some cataract surgeons utilize a laser to break up the cataract, but it still has to be removed using suction. Once the lens is removed, an intraocular lens implant is placed in the capsular bag that previously held the crystalline lens. This capsule sometimes clouds over and is often termed a secondary cataract (more technically, it is a posterior capsule opacity). A yttrium:aluminum:garnet (YAG) laser can be used to break an opening in the capsule, which is how the rumor got started that lasers can remove cataracts.
- Myth #11: Wearing glasses will make your eyes worse. Fact: Having clear vision does not worsen the eyes; however, there are two things that frequently happen that make this myth seem

plausible: (1) The perception of sight changes when you can actually compare blurred and clear vision. For example, if you cannot recall seeing clearly, especially if your vision gradually gets worse, you will think your vision is not bad. However, once you put on glasses to see clearly, the once "not too bad" vision by comparison is revealed to be blurry. (2) Eyes that get to the point of needing glasses for clear vision are often in a progressive state anyway and will therefore continue to get worse for a period of time.

- Myth #12: People become farsighted as they get older. Fact: Because the symptoms for farsightedness and mid-life presbyopia are the same (loss of ability to see close up), some think they are the same thing. However, hyperopia is usually due to a short eye length and present at birth; presbyopia is loss of the ability to focus up close as we age.
- Myth #13: Eye color changes depending on the color of your clothing. Fact: The color of the eyes does not actually change, but our perception of their color may change. It is much like placing a particular color of matting around a photograph to help "draw out" some of the colors in the picture.
- Myth #14: Eating carrots will make your vision better. Fact: The vitamin A that is found in carrots will not make blurry vision clear. It will, however, improve night vision if the person has a vitamin A deficiency.
- Myth #15: 20/20 is perfect vision. Fact: 20/20 is considered normal, average vision. The designation means that the eye can recognize a certain-sized image from 20 feet away. Many eyes are capable of vision better than 20/20 (ie, 20/15 or sometimes even 20/10), so it would be inappropriate to consider 20/20 "perfect" because then 20/15 is better than perfect.
- Myth #16: People with impaired vision develop better hearing and other senses than normal. Fact: When vision is not utilized, we depend on our other senses more and pay more attention to them, but they do not actually grow sharper. A lot of people will close their eyes when they are trying to concentrate on something else (listening, thinking, feeling, etc) to avoid the distractions of vision.

Chapter 2

Embryology and Eye Development

Tammy Langley, COT

Janice K. Ledford, COMT

KEY POINTS

- The eyes begin developing during the second week of pregnancy.
- The process of ocular formation is largely a product of different cell growth rates, as well as cellular specialization as development takes place.
- The eye begins as a thickened area called the optic primordium, becomes the optic groove, then invaginates (folds in) to form the optic vesicle. The optic vesicle is later pushed outward to develop the optic cup, from which the individual structures of the eye will arise.
- The optic cup predetermines the size and shape of the orbit. Postnatal growth of the orbit coincides with growth of the globe.
- Eyelids are fused together at first, then separate during the fifth through seventh months.
- Most babies are hyperopic at birth.

Is there anything more wondrous than a baby being formed in its mother's womb? The incredible chain of events that takes place to result in a newborn child is nothing short of a miracle. As we begin learning about the parts and functions of the eye, let us first take a look at how some of them are put together. (*Note*: This subject is very complex and has been simplified here.)

Three Primary Layers

The developing embryo has three primary germ layers: the ectoderm (outer layer), mesoderm (middle layer), and endoderm (inner layer). (Used this way, a *germ* is the earliest form of any structure.) The surface ectoderm, the neural ectoderm and neural crest (which both arise from the surface ectoderm), as well as the mesoderm are all important to the development of the eye (Table 2-1). The surface ectoderm is the source of development for the lens, lacrimal gland, corneal epithelium, epidermis of the lids, and conjunctiva. The neural ectoderm contributes to the development of the iris muscles, retinal pigment epithelium (RPE), and optic nerve fibers. The neural crest, via mesenchyme (embryonic connective tissue), gives many of the connective tissues and adnexal structures of the eye the fibrous elements they need to develop. Finally, the mesoderm is a major contributing factor to the development of the extraocular muscles (EOMs).

Ocular Formation

The process of ocular formation is largely a product of different cell growth rates, as well as cellular specialization (as development takes place). In addition, one event often seems to trigger another (ie, formation of the optic vesicle triggers the formation of the lens).

The Beginning

The eyes begin to appear during the second week of pregnancy (Table 2-2). The development of the eye occurs alongside the differentiating of the central nervous system. The eye starts as a thickened area called the optic primordium. Initially, the eyes look like shallow grooves. These optic grooves first appear on both sides of the embryonic head. During weeks 7 through 10, the eyes gradually move toward the middle of the baby's face. By 13 weeks, the eyes settle into their permanent position.

Week 3

During week 3, the optic grooves become pocket-like structures called optic vesicles. During this time, a primitive blood vessel known as the hyaloid artery forms, which will nourish the forming lens and retina. Around the 24th day of growth, the optic vesicles are pushed outward toward the surface. The connections between the vesicles and the forebrain stretch and narrow, forming the optic stalks. As the optic vesicles grow, they buckle to form the optic cup (from which the individual structures of the eye will develop). The cup fuses with the stalk and then fills with mesenchyme. The optic nerve forms as the optic stalk is ingrown with nerve fibers.

The Lens

As early as the 27th day, lens growth can be detected as a thickened area of the surface epithelial cells. This forming lens is supplied by the hyaloid artery. The early lens is tightly adhered

Table 2-1

Origin of Ocular Structures

Embryonic Tissue ⟶ Forms ⟶	Ocular Structures
Neural ectoderm	Retinal pigment epithelium Retina Iris muscles Optic nerve fibers
Surface ectoderm	Lens Corneal epithelium Lacrimal gland Epidermis of lids Epithelium of conjunctiva Epithelium of miscellaneous glands
Neural crest	Intraocular connective tissue Corneal endothelium Ciliary muscle Vitreous Orbital tissues: orbital nerves cartilage bone
Mesoderm	Extraocular muscles Endothelium of blood vessels

Table 2-2

Gestational Development of Ocular Structures

Gestation Month(s)	Embryologic Event
0 to 1	Formation of the optic pit, optic stalk, optic vesicle, and optic cup Lens begins forming Primary vitreous is present
1 to 2	Lens separates from optic cup Cornea forms: epithelium and endothelium Sclera begins forming anteriorly Iris tissues fuse Orbit begins forming Anterior chamber begins forming Pupil forms Secondary vitreous is present Eyelids form and fuse Eyebrows form Extraocular muscles begin to form Nasolacrimal drainage system begins to form Optic nerve fibers present in stalk
3	Eyes positioned in center of face Lens is 2 mm in diameter Descemet's membrane forms Sclera surrounds optic nerve Optic cup pushes forward Tertiary vitreous is present

(continued)

Table 2-2 (continued)

Gestational Development of Ocular Structures

Gestation Month(s)	Embryologic Event
4	Ciliary muscle begins to form Precursors of photoreceptors present Primitive retinal vasculature present Vitreous fully formed Zonules begin to form Schlemm's canal forms
5	Pupillary membrane disappears Bowman's membrane forms Corneal nerve endings present Sphincter muscle begins to form Macula begins to differentiate Lids begin to separate
6	Dilator muscle forms Retinal layers fully formed Aqueous begins to form
7	Lids fully separated Eyelashes present
8	Lens is 6 mm in diameter Hyaloid artery degenerates Nasolacrimal cord hollows out Pupillary membrane atrophies

to the optic vesicle, a feature that helps ensure the alignment of the lens along the optic axis. Around day 33, the lens separates from the optic cup and becomes a single entity. The optic cup stimulates epithelial cells to change into lens fibers. Once the primary and secondary fiber layers are formed, lens cells continue to form within the capsule. When these cells meet and blend, a line (called a suture line) is formed. One suture line is shaped like a Y and the other like an upside-down Y. These suture lines are sometimes visible in the mature lens. The lens grows more dense as formation progresses. The diameter of the lens is about 2 mm at 12 weeks gestation. It grows to approximately 6 mm by week 35. By the time the baby is born, the lens is almost adult-sized. It is fairly spherical at birth and continues to grow throughout life.

The Cornea

Corneal development is triggered around the 33rd day by the separation of the lens from the optic cup. At first, the cornea is nothing more than a basal membrane covered by one or two layers of epithelium. During the next week, the endothelium begins to arise, and will assume its single-cell structure by 3 months. The stroma develops next (between the epithelium and endothelium), arising from the neural crest. Descemet's membrane is first detectable around the third month. At this time, all of the corneal components are present (with the exception of Bowman's membrane, which forms at 5 months gestation).

The fetal cornea is not transparent. Because of its high hydration, the developing cornea is translucent. As the tissues mature, the water content is reduced and the cornea eventually becomes clear. Corneal nerve endings are present by the fifth month. The diameter of the cornea at birth is dependent on the size of the retinal cup. If the whole eye is smaller than normal, the cornea will be smaller as well, although all of the components will be present in proper proportions.

The Sclera

The sclera first begins to form anteriorly from mesenchyme at the limbus (at the future insertion point of the rectus muscles) around week 7, then progresses posteriorly. It completely surrounds the optic nerve by 12 weeks.

The Iris and Pupil

As growth occurs during days 30 to 35, the tissues that will form the iris fuse. If fusion is not complete, a coloboma (a gap in the iris's circular structure) occurs. The sphincter muscle develops around 5 months and the dilator muscle after month 6. Iris pigmentation generally occurs after birth. A shallow anterior chamber begins to form during week 7. By the time of a full-term birth, the angle structures are ready to drain aqueous. The ciliary muscle forms during the fourth month. By week 9 the pupil forms, but it is covered by a pupillary membrane until the fifth month.

The Retina

The tissues that will become the retina are present in the optic pit at 3 weeks. During the fourth month, the precursors of the photoreceptors develop. This is also when primitive retinal blood vessels begin to appear. The macula begins to form at midgestation, but its development is not complete until the sixth postnatal month. The retina's final formation is complete around 6 months (prenatal). The vitreous forms in three stages beginning at week 3 and continuing through the fourth month. The hyaloid artery passes through the vitreous and gives rise to the central retinal artery (CRA). The hyaloid artery is no longer needed by 8 months and undergoes degeneration. Sometimes a remnant of the hyaloid is visible on the back surface of the lens in the adult eye (Mittendorf's dot).

The Eyelids

Eyelids are detectable at the beginning of the second month. By the 11th week, they have grown to cover most of the eye's surface. The eyelids gradually fuse together and remain that way for a few months, protecting the developing eyes. While the eyelids are fused, the conjunctival sac lies over the front of the cornea. The connective tissue and tarsal plates are formed from the lids. The orbicularis oculi muscle is formed and is supplied by CN VII. The lids slowly begin to separate by about the fifth month of development. Separation is completed by the baby's seventh month of development. During the 12th through the 14th weeks, the eyebrows can be seen. By 22 weeks, the eyelids and eyebrows are very well formed. Eyelashes are present at 28 weeks.

The Extraocular Muscles

The EOMs begin to develop around week 4. The orbit begins to develop around weeks 6 through 8. It is important to note that the optic cup forms prior to this and predetermines the size and shape of the orbit. Postnatal growth of the orbit coincides with the growth of the globe;

thus, if the globe is abnormally small, the orbit remains small as well. While the eye itself reaches full size early (between 2 to 3 years of age), the orbit may not reach its full adult size until 16 years.

The Nasolacrimal System

The nasolacrimal drainage system begins forming by week 6. It arises as a solid cord of epithelial cells that is buried in the developing facial structures. The cord becomes hollow just before or just after birth. (If the cord is not completely hollowed out at birth [congenital nasolacrimal duct obstruction], tears will not be able to drain properly. The system may be opened via massage or probing.) The lacrimal glands arise from the conjunctival epithelium. They are not functional at birth, and reflex tears do not begin to accompany crying until around 3 months.

Eye Growth

The weight of the eyeball is 15 mg at 10 weeks gestation. This more than doubles over the next 2 weeks. There is a big leap between 5.5 and 6 months, when the eye grows from 269 mg to 663 mg. The eye weighs 1170 mg at 8 months . By the end of a full-term birth, the eye's weight has reached over 2800 mg.

Evaluation of the Fetal Eye

Ultrasound, *magnetic resonance imaging* (*MRI*) (difficult due to fetal movement), and *radiography* (rarely used) can give some visual information about ocular structure and facial features. *Embryoscopy* (first trimester) and *fetoscopy* (second trimester) are invasive procedures that allow direct visualization; ultrasound is generally preferred. *Evaluation of amniotic fluid* collected via amniocentesis and tissue obtained by chorionic villus sampling can reveal genetic disorders that may have ocular effects (ie, albinism, Down syndrome, etc).

Development After Birth

The eyeball grows very quickly during the first few years after birth. Growth slows for several years but then speeds up again at puberty. The infant's cornea, which is flatter than an adult's, reaches adult size by age 2. Astigmatism is common in infancy but decreases after a few years. The iris usually darkens in coloration during the first 2 years. The lens material of the infant is soft and putty-like, yielding great accommodative power. As the lens grows throughout life it lays down more fibers, becoming denser and less elastic (see Chapter 8). In addition, the neonatal lens is more spherical in shape; the adult lens is flatter.

Most babies are hyperopic at birth because of the eye's short axial length. Extreme hyperopia is negated by the nearly spherical lens of the infant. Hyperopia is usually self-corrected as the child grows and the eye increases in length. Because the lens also flattens as the eye's axial length increases, myopia is usually offset (initially) for most children.

What Newborns Can See

A newborn baby can see light and will close his or her eyes to bright light. Most newborns will exhibit a jerky following response to a target (a human face is preferred). There is poorly controlled eye movement, and intermittent eye deviations may be present. These conditions usually phase out by around the fourth month of life, and fixation becomes increasingly sharper. The visual acuity of a 2-month-old child is estimated to be around 20/400. This rises to 20/100 at 6 months, 20/50 at 1 year, and 20/20 by 3 years.

Glossary of Common Disorders

albinism: A genetic disorder in which there is a deficiency or absence of pigment. In the eye, there is a lack of skin, iris, and retinal pigment.

aniridia: Absence of the iris; in congenital cases there is usually a hereditary component.

coloboma: A developmental defect in which parts of an embryonic tissue do not properly fuse together; in the eye this can occur in the lid, iris, choroid, and/or retina and is usually seen in the lower quadrant of these structures.

congenital cataract: A lens opacity present at birth or shortly thereafter; there may be a hereditary factor.

Mittendorf's dot: A tiny opacity on the lens indicating where the hyaloid artery was attached during fetal development.

nasolacrimal obstruction (in infants): Condition in which the fetal membrane obscuring the nasolacrimal duct fails to dissolve, creating stenosis and leading to infection; symptoms are excessive tears, matter, and possibly tenderness and swelling in the nasolacrimal area.

retinitis pigmentosa: A genetic disorder in which the retina atrophies; there is loss of night, then peripheral, and finally central vision.

retinoblastoma: A genetic mutation in which a malignant tumor arises from the retinal cells of an embryo; usually develops by 3 years of age.

retinopathy of prematurity: Condition associated with the use of oxygen in premature infants, which causes an abnormal proliferation of the retinal blood vessels.

Chapter 3

The Bony Orbit

Sheila Coyne Nemeth, COMT
Carolyn Shea, COMT
Mark Schluter, MD

KEY POINTS

- The bony orbit contains the globe, fat, fascia (supportive tissues), blood vessels, and extraocular muscles (EOMs).
- The orbit serves as a protective housing for the globe and as a framework for the attachments of the EOMs.
- The seven bones that comprise the orbit are the frontal, sphenoid, zygomat, maxilla, ethmoid, lacrimal, and palatine.
- The orbit has a roof, a floor, and lateral and medial walls. The floor of the orbit is comprised mostly of thin maxillary bone, which is sometimes broken from the pressure of blunt trauma (blow-out fracture).
- The thinness of the ethmoid bone, located in the medial orbital wall, makes it susceptible to erosions from sinusitis originating from the ethmoid sinuses. Infections from the ethmoid sinuses can enter the orbital cavity and move into the brain via the orbital veins.

The globe is contained within the bony cavity of the skull known as the orbit. In addition to the eyeball, the orbit contains fat, fascia (supportive tissues), vessels, and EOMs. The orbits are not round but are shaped more like a square-based cone with the apex of the cone pointing toward the back of the head and angled slightly inward (medially).

The orbit serves as the "protective housing" of the fragile globe. The globe requires an environment with great stability, which the strong orbital rim supplies. The orbit also serves as part of the framework for the origins of the EOMs, as they insert into the globe at specific anatomical locations.

The Bones and Walls of the Orbit

The seven bones that comprise the orbit are the frontal, sphenoid, zygomat, maxilla, ethmoid, lacrimal, and palatine. In order to remember these, make up a sentence using the first letter of each bone, such as "Fred and Sam gave Zelda Many Extra Lumps of Potatoes." Then think of the orbit as having a roof, a floor, a lateral wall (temporal) and a medial wall (nasal) (Figure 3-1). Many of the bones that comprise these walls are also walls of the paranasal sinuses (Figure 3-2).

The Roof

The roof of the orbit is primarily comprised of the frontal bone and its frontal sinus. The lateral aspect of this bone contains a depression for the lacrimal gland.

The Floor

The orbital floor is composed of three bones: the maxilla, the zygomat, and the palatine bones—but primarily the maxillary bone. During blunt trauma, such as from a fist-in-the-eye fight, the strong rim (or margin) of the orbit remains intact. However, the concussive forces from such a blow create a pressure within the orbit, so the pressure build-up seeks the weakest spot to release its tension, which is usually the orbital floor. Classically, this fracture is known as a blow-out fracture. (The medial wall is the next most common fracture site.)

The Lateral Wall

The lateral wall is the strongest wall of the orbit. It is primarily composed of the zygomatic bone (laterally) and sphenoid wing (posteriorly). If this wall fractures from blunt trauma, it usually fractures along two suture lines (the zygomaticofrontal and the zygomaticomaxillary), resulting in a tripod fracture. Because the zygoma is part of a moving joint (the jaw), it must be rewired surgically if unstable.

The Medial Wall

The medial wall of the orbit is made up of the maxilla, lacrimal, ethmoid, and sphenoid bones. The exceeding thinness of the ethmoid bone makes it as breakable as an eggshell. The ethmoid sinus lies within the ethmoid bone. Because the medial orbital wall is so thin, erosions or perforations can occur secondary to sinus infections. If perforations occur, infections from the ethmoid sinuses can enter the orbital cavity. Orbital infections may actually move into the brain via the orbital veins.

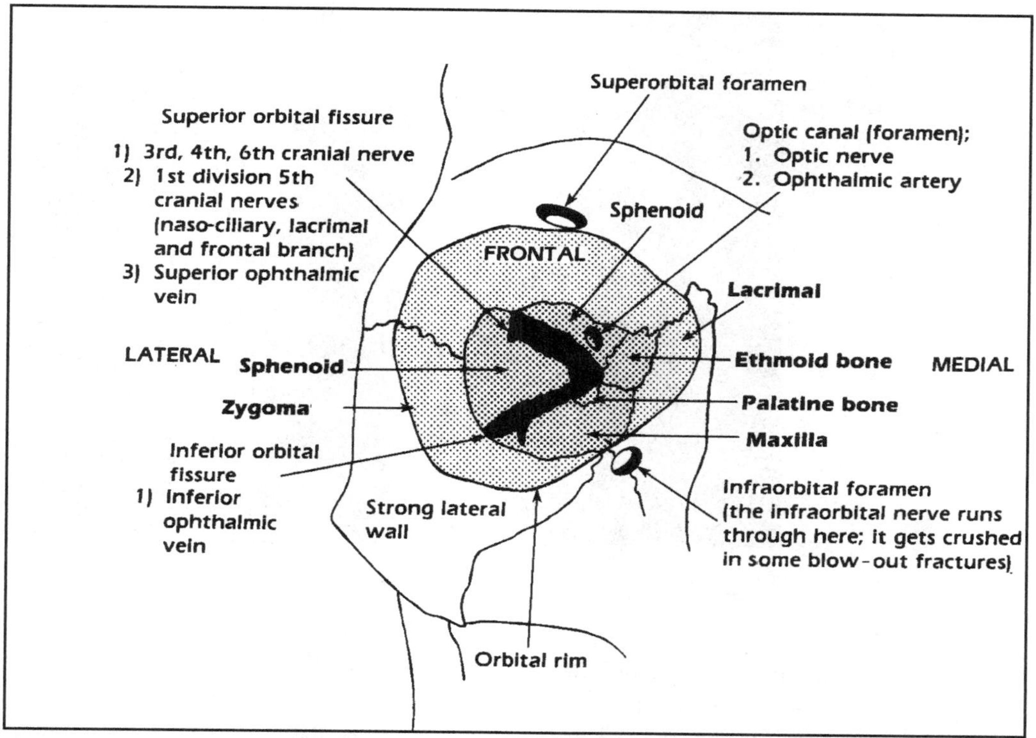

Figure 3-1. Bones and openings in the orbit. (Reprinted with permission from Nemeth SC, Shea CA. *Medical Sciences for the Ophthalmic Assistant*. Thorofare, NJ: SLACK Incorporated; 1988.)

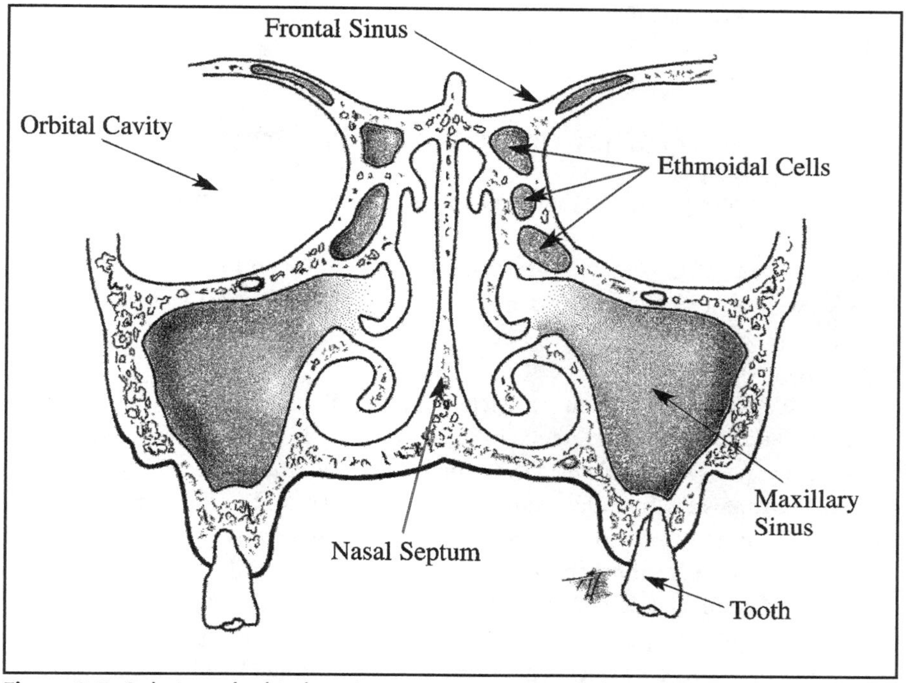

Figure 3-2. Relation of orbital cavity to sinuses. (Drawing by Ana Edwards.)

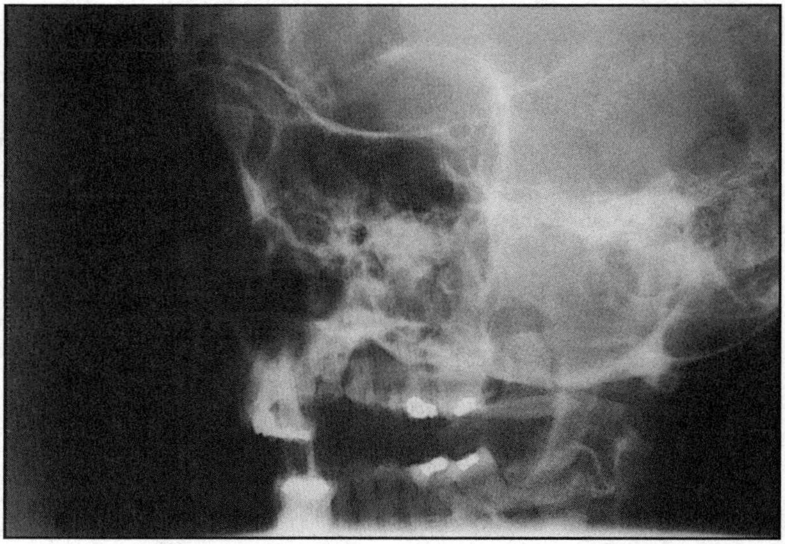

Figure 3-3. X-ray showing the orbits. (X-ray courtesy of Melissa Cabe RT(R) and Jim Ledford, PA-C. Reprinted with permission from Bittinger M. *General Medical Knowledge for Eyecare Paraprofessionals.* Thorofare, NJ: SLACK Incorporated; 1999.)

Orbital Openings

There are several important openings into the orbit (see Figure 3-1).

- The optic foremen (hole) is located at the apex of the orbit and contains the optic nerve, or cranial nerve II. This is also known as the optic canal. The ophthalmic and sympathetic nerves run through this canal as well.
- The fissure (crack) just superior and lateral to the optic canal is the superior orbital fissure, through which many cranial nerves pass (see Figure 3-1). The lower fissure is appropriately termed the inferior orbital fissure.

Evaluation of the Bony Orbit

In evaluating the orbit for trauma, inflammation, or tumors, a variety of imaging studies can be performed.

Conventional *x-ray films* (Figure 3-3) are helpful in confirming the presence of metallic foreign bodies, as well as other situations where there is significant contrast in anatomical structures adjacent to each other (ie, orbital soft tissue in a normally clear sinus or displaced fractures of some bony elements).

X-rays are taken with the beam at a predetermined angle in order to optimize viewing of the desired anatomy and to avoid interference by other structures. A common posteroanterior view, called the Waters view, is obtained when the patient's neck is extended and only the chin touches the film. It demonstrates the maxillary sinuses and the orbital roof and is useful when blow-out fractures or frontal sinus tumors are suspected. The Caldwell view is a more direct posteroanterior view (ie, the x-rays pass through the back of the head toward the front), with the forehead and nose touching the film. It demonstrates the superior and lateral orbital rims.

Computerized axial tomography (CT scans) uses computer processed x-rays taken at multiple angles to create "slices" of an object. This process allows for much more anatomic detail to be obtained. Various soft tissues can be characterized by their density (fat, muscle, brain, etc) and

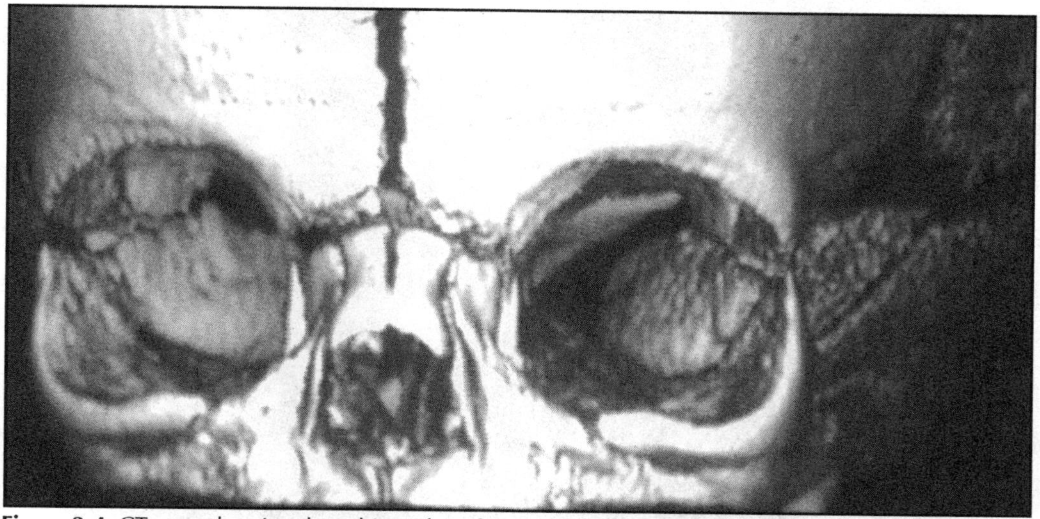

Figure 3-4. CT scan showing the orbits. (Photo by Mark Greenwald, University of Tennessee-Memphis. Reprinted with permission from Bittinger M. *General Medical Knowledge for Eyecare Paraprofessionals.* Thorofare, NJ: SLACK Incorporated; 1999.)

their relationships to each other and to bony structures (Figure 3-4). Fractures, foreign bodies, tumor margins, and inflammatory processes can be clearly identified and precisely localized with CT. Contrast enhancement by intravenous injection of an iodine-containing dye assists in the visualization of neoplasms and inflammatory tissue. This is because vessels in those areas tend to leak, leading to dye accumulation.

Magnetic resonance imaging (MRI) utilizes the magnetic properties of the hydrogen nucleus when it is excited by radiofrequency radiation in the presence of a strong magnetic field. These "jazzed-up" hydrogen nuclei emit signals, and the MRI computer analyzes these signals and processes them into a photo image (Figure 3-5).

MRI provides better definition of tissues and fluids than does the CT. It is therefore superior in differentiating tissues (such as white and gray matter) and posterior fossa anatomy. However, it does not provide adequate bone views for evaluation of fractures and is contraindicated in the presence of metallic foreign bodies or hardware.

A coronal scan of the orbit with MRI can be useful for examining the degree of inflammation of the EOMs in dysthyroid ophthalmopathy (Graves' disease), as each muscle can be clearly distinguished and assessed.

In *ultrasonography* (echography), high frequency sound waves are projected into the eye and orbit. These waves reflect off of surfaces or areas where tissue density suddenly changes. The echoes can be displayed as a real time cross-sectional image (B-mode) of the eye and orbit (Figure 3-6). Clinically, ultrasonography is very useful in determining posterior segment anatomy in the presence of poor or opaque media (ie, cataract, blood, or anterior segment disorganization). Ultrasonography also provides valuable information on ocular mass lesions, such as their size, height, and internal characteristics (internal reflectivity).

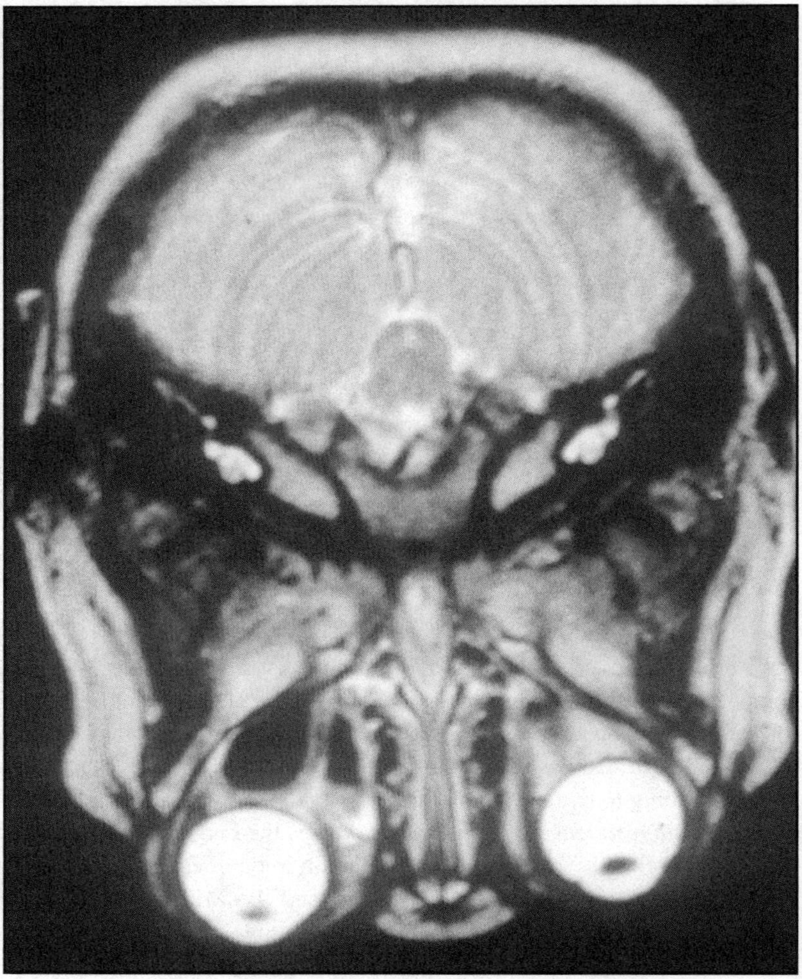

Figure 3-5. An MRI showing the orbits. (Photo by Mark Greenwald, University of Tennessee-Memphis. Reprinted with permission from Bittinger M. *General Medical Knowledge for Eyecare Paraprofessionals*. Thorofare, NJ: SLACK Incorporated; 1999.)

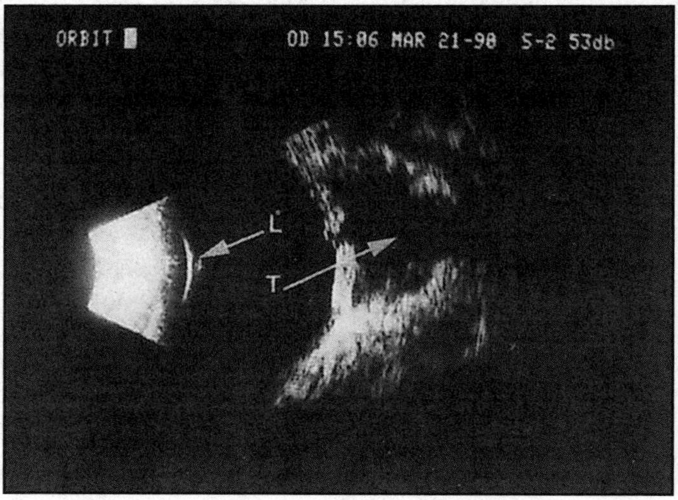

Figure 3-6. B-scan of the orbit showing the lens (L) and an orbital tumor (T). (Reprinted with permission from Kendall CJ. *Ophthalmic Echography*. Thorofare, NJ: SLACK Incorporated; 1990.)

Glossary of Common Disorders

blow-out fracture: Fracture of the orbit, usually from blunt trauma; strong concussive forces create pressure within the orbit, causing a fracture to the orbital floor. If the soft tissue of the orbit is entrapped in the fracture, double vision (especially in upgaze) and numbness on the medial side of the affected cheek can occur.

sinusitis: Infection/inflammation of the sinuses surrounding the orbits; prolonged sinusitis may erode the thin ethmoid bone (located in the medial orbital wall), allowing infection to enter the orbital cavity which can then lead to the brain via the orbital veins.

tripod fracture: Fracture to the lateral wall of the orbit along two suture lines; it can affect the jaw and its movement.

Chapter 4

Eyebrows, Eyelids, and the Lacrimal System

Tammy Langley, COT

Janice K. Ledford, COMT

KEY POINTS

- Muscles of facial expression move the eyebrows.
- The eyelids protect the eye from trauma, dryness, and too much light.
- The appearance of the external eye can vary from race to race and all are simply variations of normal.
- The gray line is often used as a landmark for eyelid surgery.
- The two divisions of the lacrimal system are the secretory system for the delivery of the tears and the excretory system for disposal of the tears.
- A normal tear film consist of three layers: mucin, water, and oil (lipid).

The Eyebrows

The eyebrows (Figure 4-1) are positioned at the intersection of the forehead and the upper lid. The hairs are usually thick and lie horizontally. The brows are moved by the muscles of facial expression. Contraction of the frontalis muscle raises the eyebrows. Contracting the orbital sections of orbicularis oculi lowers the eyebrows, and contracting the corrugator supercilia muscle draws the eyebrows together medially. These muscles are all supplied by the seventh cranial nerve (CN VII).

The Eyelids

The eyelids (see Figure 4-1) protect the eye from trauma, dryness, and too much light. They also assist with lubrication of the anterior surface of the eye by blinking. The upper eyelids are larger and more moveable than the lower eyelids. The eyelids meet at the medial and lateral angles (also known as canthi; singular is canthus). The opening between the eyelids is known as the palpebral fissure. This opening normally ranges from 8 mm to 11 mm. When the eyelids are wide open, the average of the lateral fissure angle is 60 degrees; medially the fissure is rounded. In Asian people, the medial angle is overlapped by a vertical skin fold called the epicanthus. The appearance of the external eye can vary from race to race, and all are simply variations of normal.

Young children sometimes have a prominent epicanthal fold, causing them to appear esotropic (the eye or eyes seem to turn inward, making the child look "cross-eyed") (Figure 4-2). Most infants lose this cross-eyed appearance as they grow; their facial structure "stretches out" and the epicanthus disappears.

When the eye is closed, the entire cornea should be covered by the eyelid. If the lids do not close completely, the condition is termed *lagophthalmos*. When looking straight ahead with the eye open, the upper lid rests just below the superior margin of the cornea. If the eyelid is lower than this, it is referred to as *ptosis*. The lower lid should cover 1 mm to 2 mm of the inferior cornea. If the cornea is exposed inferiorly to the point that sclera is visible, we say that the patient has scleral show. The lower lid elevates just slightly when the eye is closed.

The lateral angle of the eyelid rests flush against the eye, while the medial angle is approximately 6 mm from the eye.

The medial angle has a small pink elevation called the caruncle. The caruncle has small hairs that function as a trap for secretions in the corner of the eye, as well as sebaceous glands that contribute oil to the tear film. The soft, half-moon fold of tissue next to the caruncle is the semilunaris plica. The plica represents the junction of the bulbar conjunctiva and muscle tissue.

The eyelid margin is 2 mm thick and approximately 30 mm long. The lateral portion of each lid is squared off like a ledge, while the medial area is slightly rounded. The eyelashes are on the anterior border of the eyelid margins. The upper lid's lashes are curved slightly upward, and the lower lashes curve down. The lashes are two or three rows thick. They are usually their longest and most curled during childhood.

If you pull the lower lid down and look medially, you will see a peaked area of the lid with a small opening in the center. This opening is the punctum. The average size of this opening is 0.3 mm, and its function is to allow tears to drain off of the eye. There is a punctum in each of the four eyelids.

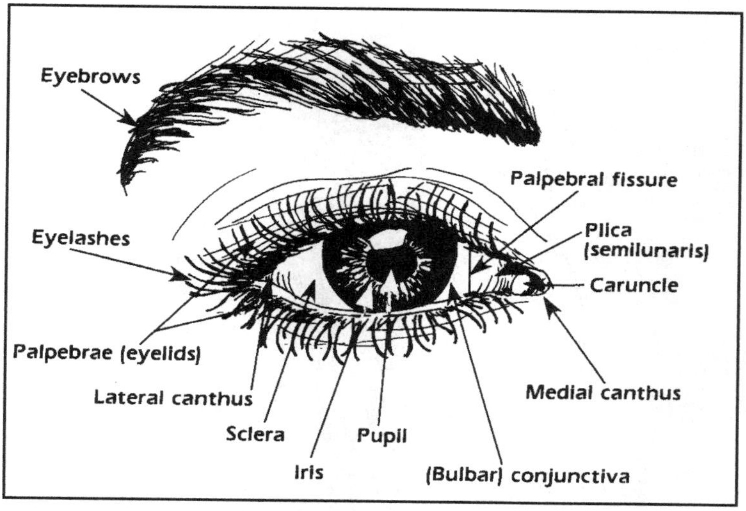

Figure 4-1. External eye. (Reprinted with permission from Nemeth SC, Shea CA. *Medical Sciences for the Ophthalmic Assistant.* Thorofare, NJ: SLACK Incorporated; 1988.)

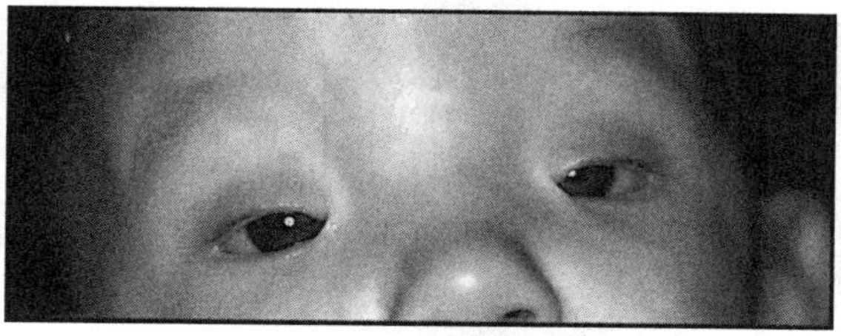

Figure 4-2. Epicanthal folds. (Photo by Mark Greenwald, University of Tennessee—Memphis.)

If the eyelid is inverted, you can see the tarsal glands on the inner surface. They are more commonly known as meibomian glands and appear as yellowish lines. These glands open onto the lid margin. Sometimes a slight groove or gray line can be distinguished between the eyelashes and the openings of the meibomian glands (Figure 4-3). This line is often used by surgeons as a demarcation between the anterior side of the eyelid (formed by skin and muscle) and the posterior side of the eyelid (formed by the tarsus and conjunctiva).

Evaluation of the Lids and Brows

The lids and brows are best observed using the *slit lamp microscope*. Diffuse or direct lighting may be used, and photographs may be taken as well. External photography (ie, not taken at the slit lamp) is often used to document abnormalities. If the slit lamp has a ruler built into the reticule, lesions may be measured at the microscope as well. The width of the fissures or size of lesions can also be measured using a *millimeter rule* or *calipers*. *Cytology* (including Gram and Giemsa staining) and cultures may be used to identify microorganisms from lesions. The width of the fissures can also be measured using a *millimeter rule* or *calipers*.

The Lacrimal System

The lacrimal system consists of several different entities working together to provide lubrication to the eye. The major structures of the system include the lacrimal gland, the lacrimal canaliculi, the lacrimal sac, and the nasolacrimal duct (Figure 4-4). The two divisions of the

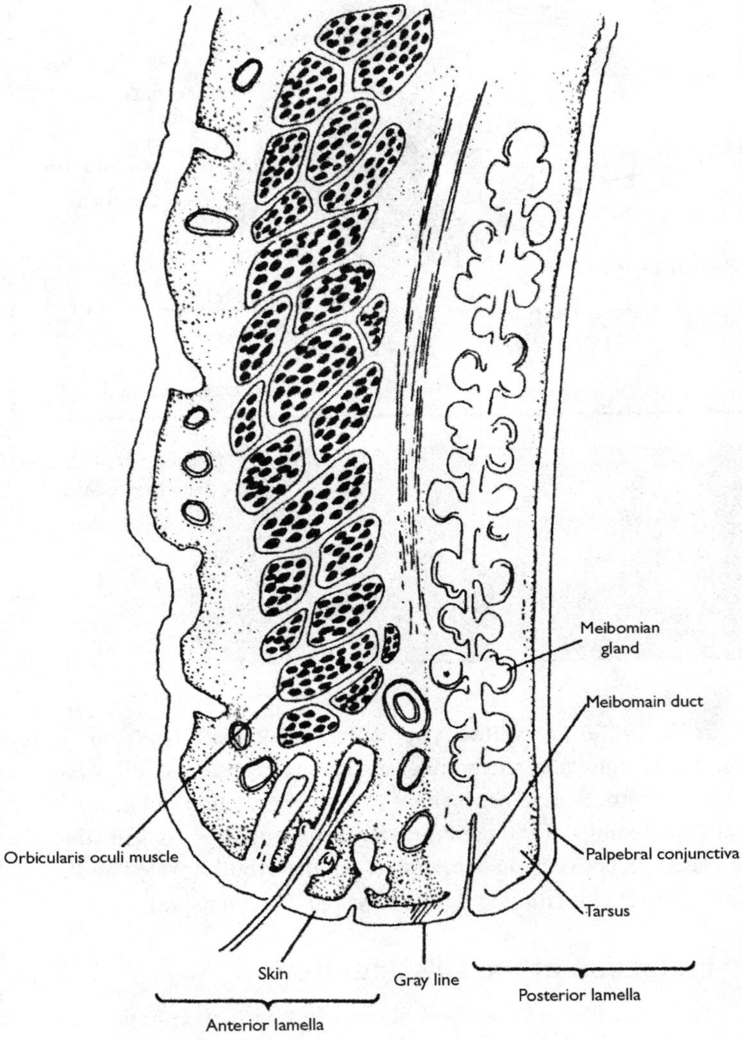

Figure 4-3. Section of the upper lid. (Reprinted with permission from Meltzer MA. *Ophthalmic Plastic Surgery for the General Ophthalmologist.* Baltimore, MD: Williams and Wilkins; 1979.)

lacrimal system are the secretory system, which delivers the tears, and the excretory system, which disposes of the tears.

Secretory System

The composition of the tear film is vital to the lubrication of the cornea and external globe. A normal tear film consists of three layers: the inner mucus layer (mucin), the intermediate aqueous (watery) layer, and the outer oily (lipid) layer. Only when all three ingredients are present in the correct balance does the cornea receive proper nutrients and protection. In dry eye conditions, it is often the case that the balance of the three layers has been disturbed.

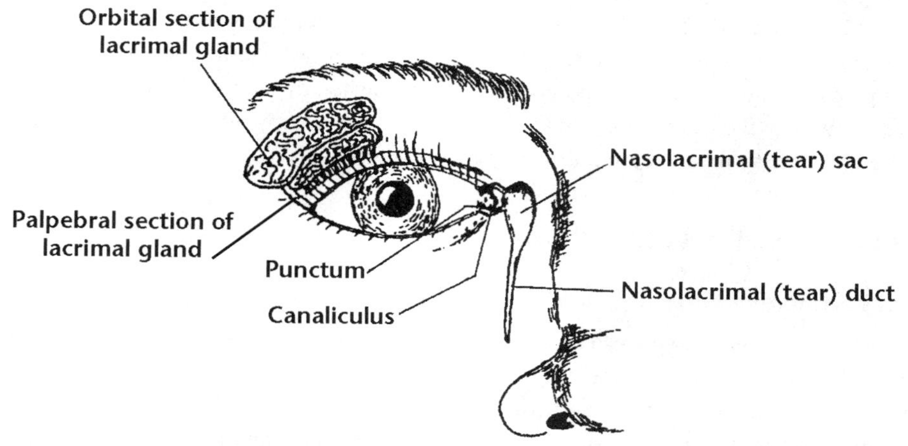

Figure 4-4. The nasolacrimal system. (Drawing by Holly Smith. Reprinted with permission from Gayton JL, Ledford JR. *The Crystal Clear Guide to Sight for Life.* Lancaster, PA: Starburst Publishers; 1996.)

The mucin layer contacts the tissues directly, filling in any microscopic irregularities on the cornea. This is important in the creation of a smooth refractive surface, as well as to wet the surface of the cornea. (Because of the hydrophobic nature of the corneal epithelium, it cannot be moistened well by the water layer alone.) The watery layer, the major component of tears, contains proteins and salts and overlies the mucin. On top of the watery layer is the oil (lipid) layer. The oil helps slow the evaporation of the tears off the eye's surface. Immunoglobulins are also present in the tears, helping to inhibit infection. In addition, oxygen for corneal metabolism comes largely from the tear film. The normal pH of the tears ranges from 5.20 to 8.35. The amount of tears on the eye ranges from 5 to 9 microliters.

The lacrimal gland secretes the aqueous portion of the tear film and is located superiotemporal and just posterior to the orbital rim. The lacrimal gland has two sections. The larger section is the orbital portion, and the smaller is the palpebral portion. The gland wraps around the tendon of the levator palpebrae superioris. It can be seen underneath the conjunctiva in the lateral part of the superior fornix when the eyelid is everted.

Goblet cells provide the mucin layer of the tear film. The goblet cells are found within the conjunctiva. Meibomian glands in the lids produce the oil layer of the tear film. There are some other accessory glands that help with tear secretion as well. These are the glands of Krause and Wolfring, which are located in the superior tarsal conjunctiva.

Excretory System

The punctum is the external landmark for the excretory portion of the lacrimal system. When in its proper position, the lid is inverted slightly so that the punctum contacts the globe. The tears are pumped toward the punctum during each blink. In addition, when the orbicularis muscle contracts, the lacrimal sac expands, which creates an internal pressure change. The fluid is then drawn downward through the punctum. Once the fluid has left the eye, the tears flow through the superior or inferior canaliculus. These are small tubes that originate at the punctum, coursing for 2 mm vertically and then 8 mm horizontally toward the nasal passages. There the two canaliculi meet and join at the lateral wall of the lacrimal sac. The lacrimal sac is located nasally and lies perpendicular to the canaliculi within the lacrimal fossa. Inferior to the lacrimal sac is the nasolacrimal duct (NLD). This duct is approximately 12 mm in length and opens into the nasal passages through an ostium (small opening) located beneath and lateral to the inferior turbinate. From here the tears drain into the back of the throat. (How often have your patients told you of the bad taste in their mouth after using their eye drops?)

Evaluation of the Lacrimal System

Secretory System

The *slit lamp biomicroscope* can be used to view the tear film directly. The tear lake (pooling of tears at the lower lid margin) can be fully evaluated. This may be easier if *fluorescein dye* is instilled. In addition, the tear film can be evaluated for the presence of debris or matter. An oily sheen on the tear film surface may indicate an overproduction of the lipid layer. Alternately, rose bengal stain may be used. If the stain reveals areas on the conjunctival or corneal surfaces, tear function is deficient.

The *Schirmer's tear test* is the standard of measurement for tear output. A thin strip of filter paper is placed between the lower lid and the globe for 5 minutes. After that time, the strip is removed and the length of the strip that has been wet by tears is measured with a millimeter ruler. The test can be done with or without topical anesthetic. If topical anesthetic is used, there should be 10 mm of wetting in a 5-minute test time. Less than 10 mm of wetting in that time frame indicates inadequate tear production.

The *tear break-up time (BUT)* uses the slit lamp to evaluate the wetting ability of the tear film. Fluorescein drops are first instilled. With the cobalt blue filter, the examiner looks at the patient's corneal surface through the slit lamp. The patient is asked to blink (which swabs fluorescein over the cornea) and then to keep the lids open. The examiner counts the number of seconds that pass before the tear film breaks and a dry spot appears on the cornea. In the normal tear film, BUT is 15 to 30 seconds; less than 10 seconds is considered abnormal.

Excretory System

The patency of the nasolacrimal drainage system can be evaluated via *irrigation*. The lower punctum is gently dilated after a drop of topical anesthetic is instilled. Once the opening has been stretched, a cannula (attached to a syringe filled with sterile saline solution) is gently inserted through the punctum. The syringe is slowly depressed. If the system is open, saline will flow through it and into the back of the patient's throat.

Fluorescein drops can also be used to evaluate the drainage system. Fluorescein is instilled into the eye. After a few minutes, the examiner uses a penlight (covered with a blue filter) to examine inside the patient's nostrils or the back of the patient's throat. If the system is open, fluorescein dye should be visible. In another variation of this test, fluorescein dye is injected via a cannula directly into the nasolacrimal sac. The system is patent if fluorescein is excreted when the patient blows his or her nose. One can also observe the drainage of fluorescein from the eye. First, if the dye disappears from one eye more quickly than the other, the eye with the delay probably has an obstruction. The second eye should be cleared from an open system within about 5 minutes.

The *Hornblass saccharine test* determines patency of the drainage system in each eye. Saccharine is dropped into one eye, and after several minutes chloramphenicol is dropped into the other eye. A sweet taste indicates the eye with the saccharine is open; the eye with the chloramphenicol is patent if a bitter taste is experienced.

Dacryocystography refers to any imaging of the nasolacrimal system. A contrast dacryocystography (x-ray of the drainage system) is possible if a dye that shows up on x-rays is injected into the nasolacrimal system. A *magnetic resonance imaging (MRI)* using gadolinium to provide contrast can also reveal NLD obstructions. A *computed tomography (CT)* scan may also be used to establish obstruction as well as help identify the obstruction (ie, scar tissue, tumor/growth, etc).

Alternately, *dacryoscintigraphy* utilizes a radioactive drop that is placed into the eye. Photographs are taken by a gamma camera (or nuclear scanner) with a special filter as the dye drains from the eye.

Suspected infections can be evaluated by examining discharge via *cytology* (including Gram and Giemsa staining), as well as *culturing* for microorganisms.

Glossary of Common Disorders

blepharitis: Inflammation/infection of the eyelids that can be allergic, viral, or bacterial; signs and symptoms include redness, crusting on lashes, blocked meibomian glands, itching, and lid thickening.

blepharoptosis: See ptosis.

canaliculitis: Inflammation of the canaliculus.

chalazion: Inflammation/infection of a meibomian gland.

dacryocystitis: Infection of the nasolacrimal duct.

dermatochalasis: Redundancy of tissue of the upper lids, sometimes hanging below the lid margin and affecting the superior visual field.

dry eye: Disorder in which the eye does not make enough tears or the composition of the tears is not optimal; signs and symptoms include gritty sensation and excessive tearing.

ectropion: Condition in which the lower lid lags outward, exposing the palpebral conjunctiva.

entropion: Condition in which the lower lid turns inward, causing the lashes to rub on the cornea.

epiphora: Excessive tear flow due either to overproduction of tears or insufficient drainage by the lacrimal system.

hordeolum ("sty"): Inflammation/infection of an eyelash follicle.

lacrimal obstruction: Condition in which the nasolacrimal duct is blocked; excessive tearing occurs because the tears cannot drain properly and infection may appear in the nasolacrimal system due to stenosis.

lagophthalmos*: Incomplete closure of eyelids, which may result in exposure keratitis.

ptosis (also called blepharoptosis): Drooping of the upper lid.

trichiasis: Condition in which a lash or lashes (on either lid) grow aberrantly and rub against the globe/cornea.

* These definitions are used with permission from Ledford JK, Hoffman J. *Quick Reference Dictionary of Eyecare Terminology, Fifth Edition.* Thorofare, NJ: SLACK Incorporated; 2008.

Chapter 5

Extraocular Muscles and the Globe

Carolyn Shea, COMT

Sheila Coyne Nemeth, COMT

Janice K. Ledford, COMT

KEY POINTS

- Each globe is located in the anterior portion of the orbit, near the roof and the lateral wall.
- The globe itself occupies only one-fifth of the orbital cavity.
- The globe is least protected on the lateral side.
- The globe is not round but made up of two modified spheres joined at the limbus (junction of the cornea and sclera). The cornea is the smaller "sphere" with a radius of 7.8 mm, and the larger posterior "sphere" has a radius of 17 mm.
- The globe is widest at the anterior-posterior diameter (24 mm) and flatter vertically (23 mm). Its horizontal diameter is 23.5 mm.

The Globe

The adult eyeball, or globe, measures approximately 1 inch or 2.5 cm in diameter—roughly the size of a quarter. Of the total diameter of the eye, only the anterior one-sixth is visible externally. The rest is protected by cushioning tissues and the well-designed bony orbit. (Individual structures of the globe will be covered in detail in other chapters.)

Layers of the Globe

There are several ways to divide the globe into sections. The globe can be viewed as having three separate layers (Figure 5-1), each with its own unique function. These strata are the fibrous/protective outer layer, the middle vascular/nourishing layer, and the innermost nerve/sensory layer.

The Fibrous/Protective Layer

The eye's contents are protected by the tough outer coating of the sclera. (Some references include the cornea in the protective layer as well.) The sclera is commonly known as the "white of the eye." It forms the posterior portion of the globe and contains the vitreous humor. The cornea, the anterior portion of the globe, is transparent and allows light into the eye. The junction of the cornea and sclera is known as the limbus.

It is interesting to note that the sclera and cornea are actually composed of basically the same fibrous material. The fibers of the cornea are laid out in a specific criss-cross fashion and are kept dehydrated by the corneal endothelium. These two features maintain the clarity of the cornea. If the corneal tissue becomes edematous, it turns opaque like the sclera. If an area of scleral tissue becomes dehydrated, it will become more transparent (although obviously not as clear as the cornea).

The Vascular/Nourishing Layer

The middle layer is composed of blood vessel-rich tissues that bring nourishment to the retina via the blood supply. Collectively, this layer is composed of the uvea (or uveal tract), which itself has three components: the iris, the ciliary body, and the choroid.

The uveal tract also contains the pigment melanin. The amount of pigment present is a product of genetics, thus eye color is an inherited factor. (A blue-eyed person has less pigment than a brown-eyed person.)

The Nerve/Sensory Layer

The innermost surface of the globe is the retina with its photoreceptive properties. The retina lies over the choroid and is extremely thin (although composed of nine layers itself), transparent, and delicate. The retina contains the highly specialized visual receptor cells called rods and cones (which convert light energy into nerve impulses) as well as neurons (which transmit the converted light energy through the optic nerve).

Global Divisions

The globe can also be thought of as being divided into two asymmetric cavities: the anterior and posterior segments (Figure 5-2).

The anterior segment includes the lens and the structures anterior to it. This segment is viewed anatomically as two chambers: the anterior chamber (AC) and the posterior chamber (PC). The

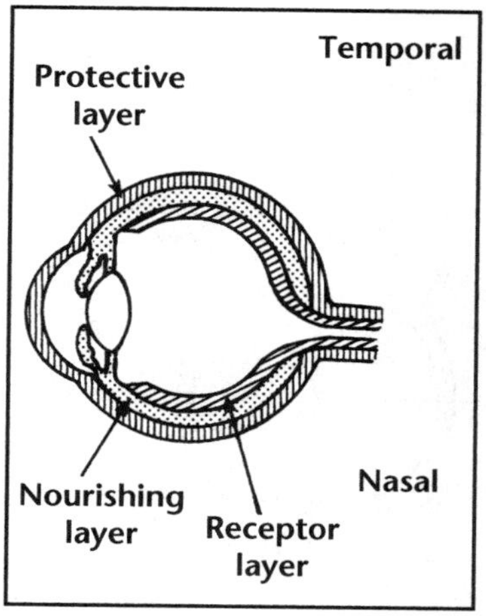

Figure 5-1. The three layers of the globe. (Reprinted with permission from Nemeth SC, Shea CA. *Medical Sciences for the Ophthalmic Assistant.* Thorofare, NJ: SLACK Incorporated; 1988.)

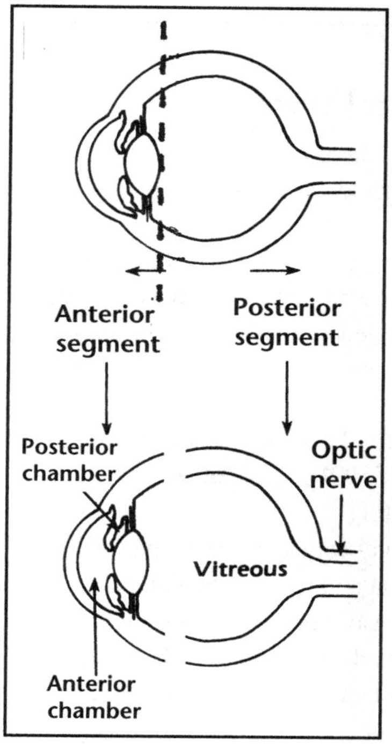

Figure 5-2. Segments and chambers of the globe. (Reprinted with permission from Nemeth SC, Shea CA. *Medical Sciences for the Ophthalmic Assistant.* Thorofare, NJ: SLACK Incorporated; 1988.)

AC is delimited by the anterior iris and posterior surface of the cornea, and is filled with aqueous humor. The PC is contained between the posterior surface of the iris and the anterior surface of the crystalline lens. The aqueous is formed here but circulates through the pupil into the hollow of the AC.

The posterior is the larger of the two segments. It begins at the posterior face of the crystalline lens and is bound peripherally by the sclera. The optic nerve (the second cranial nerve, or CN II) pierces the sclera and is part of the posterior segment. This nerve receives impulses from the retinal neurons and directs them to the brain for interpretation. If this pathway is interrupted anywhere along its route to the brain (by trauma or disease), vision will be impaired and the center for perception will receive faulty input.

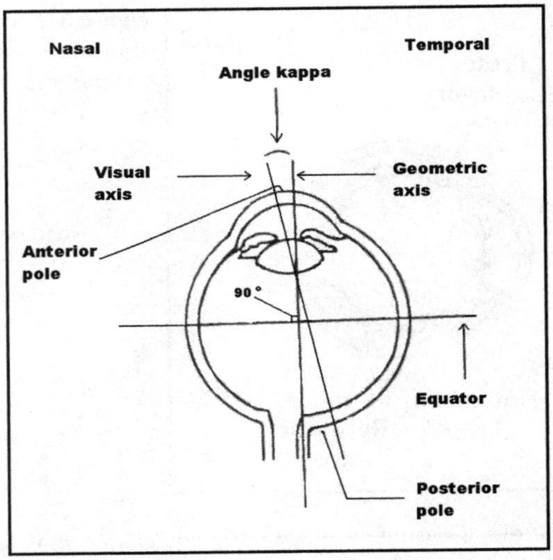

Figure 5-3. Schematic of ocular landmarks. Note that the visual axis is slightly nasal in order to intersect the fovea (area of finest central vision in the retina). The eye's equator is slightly more posterior on the temporal side due to the angle of the globe in the orbit. (Adapted from Nemeth SC, Shea CA. *Medical Sciences for the Ophthalmic Assistant.* Thorofare, NJ: SLACK Incorporated; 1988.)

Ocular Dimensions, Landmarks, and Anatomical Directions

Knowledge of several clinical dimensions and landmarks of the globe help in understanding terminology and testing procedures (Figure 5-3). For standardized ocular dimensions, refer to Chapter 15.

The normal anterior/posterior diameter of the adult eye is 24.5 mm. Clinically, this is referred to as the axial length (AL) measurement of the globe. This measurement is ascertained by an ultrasonic instrument known as an A-scan. This length is needed prior to cataract surgery to calculate the power of the intraocular lens (IOL) implant, the device which replaces the natural lens.

The average corneal diameter of the adult eye is 12.0 mm. This measurement ("white to white") is used to select the proper size of an AC IOL. (A PC IOL does not require a "size" because it fits behind the iris.) It is also used in contact lens fitting.

The *visual* axis of the globe is the line "connecting" the visual center of the retina (called the fovea) with the optical center of the refracting system (the cornea and lens). When one is measuring the axial length of the eye, one is actually attempting to measure the visual axis. This is why probe alignment is so important during A-scans. If the probe is directed toward the optic nerve (instead of the fovea), the reading will be erroneously long. This can lead to an error in IOL power selection, resulting in an unwanted postoperative refractive error.

The average AL of 24.5 mm is typical of emmetropia (no refractive error). Longer AL measurements may indicate myopia (nearsightedness), while shorter lengths may indicate hyperopia (farsightedness).

The *geometric* axis is the line that exactly bisects the eye in the anterior/posterior direction. The reflection of light on a person's cornea (the corneal reflex) is displaced slightly nasal to the true geometric center. This is because the fovea is displaced slightly temporally. The normal nasal displacement of the light reflex is known as a positive angle kappa. A large positive angle kappa can make a person appear exotropic (eye crosses out), although there is actually no manifest strabismus.

The crossing of the visual and geometric axes also creates two anatomical landmarks. The anterior pole is the central section of cornea between the two axes. The posterior pole is the

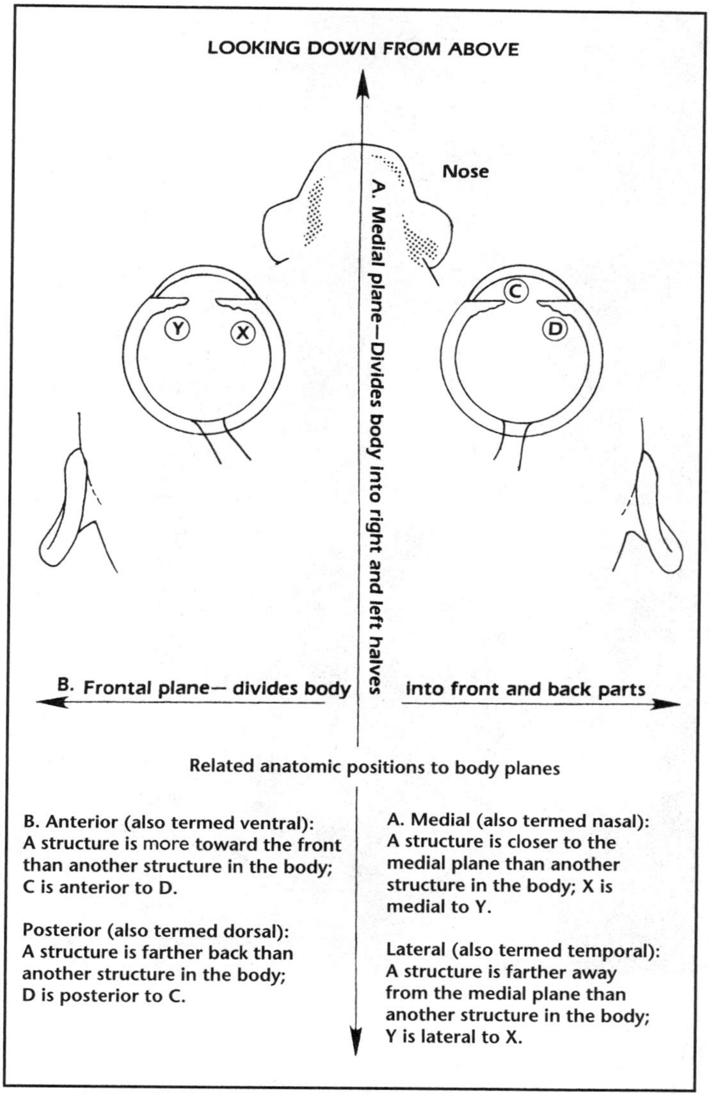

Figure 5-4. Basic anatomical directions. (Reprinted with permission from Nemeth SC, Shea CA. *Medical Sciences for the Ophthalmic Assistant.* Thorofare, NJ: SLACK Incorporated; 1988.)

portion of retina between the two axes (ie, between the optic nerve and fovea) and the superior and inferior temporal arteries. Traditionally, this encompasses approximately 6 mm of central retina.

The geometric equator of the globe is a vertically oriented circle around the eye, perpendicular to the geometric axis. There is a slight obliqueness to this equatorial line as it lies farther posterior on the temporal side than on the nasal side due to the medial location of the optic nerve. The equator is an important landmark in retinal anatomic drawings, as well as in retinal surgery. The equator lies approximately 15 mm posterior to the corneal limbus in an eye of normal AL.

A final landmark is the fundus. In ophthalmology, the fundus refers to that part of the eye's interior that lies opposite the pupil, namely the optic disc, retinal vessels, macula, and surrounding retina.

Figure 5-4 summarizes the common anatomical body planes and directions used in ocular anatomy.

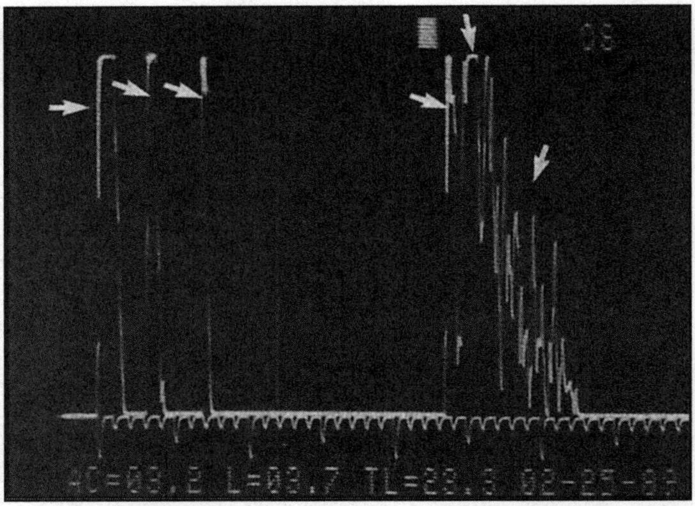

Figure 5-5. A-scan of the eye. (Reprinted with permission from Kendall CJ. *Ophthalmic Echography.* Thorofare, NJ: SLACK Incorporated; 1990.)

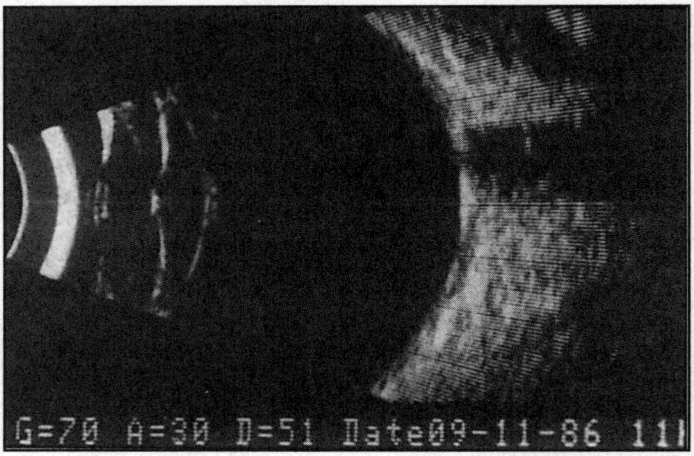

Figure 5-6. B-scan of the eye showing both corneal surfaces, both lens surfaces, retina, optic nerve, and orbital fat. (Reprinted with permission from Kendall CJ. *Ophthalmic Echography.* Thorofare, NJ: SLACK Incorporated; 1990.)

Evaluation of the Globe

There are several modalities that can be used to examine the globe as a whole.

Ultrasound (echography) utilizes sound waves to evaluate the eye. The sound waves are sent through the eye, and returning echoes are interpreted by a computer. Ultrasonic measurement of intraocular distances depends on the velocity of sound through various tissues of the eye over time, as well as the direction of the sound beam as it is sent through the eye. An *A-scan* (Figure 5-5) gives a linear read-out, usually used to provide an axial measurement of the eye's length. A B-scan (Figure 5-6) yields a two-dimensional image of the eye in real time. It is used to assess ocular tissues, especially when cloudy media prevent clear, direct visualization. In this manner, for example, one may ascertain that the retina is intact in an eye with a totally opaque crystalline lens.

Computed axial tomography (CT) is a very specific x-ray that traverses the eye section by section from many different angles (see Figure 3-4). The CT can be used to identify the extent and configuration of progressing lesions.

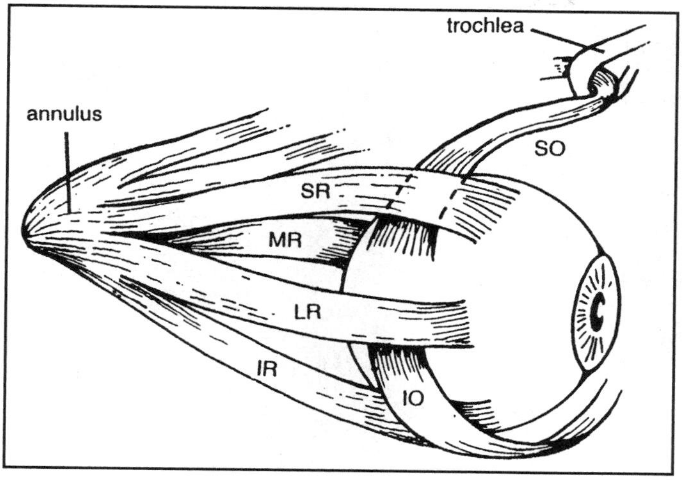

Figure 5-7. Schematic of the EOMs, side view. The four rectus muscles originate at the annulus of Zinn. (Reprinted with permission from Cassin B, ed. *Fundamentals for Ophthalmic Technical Personnel.* Philadelphia, PA: WB Saunders; 1995.)

Magnetic resonance imaging (MRI) uses a highly specialized magnet and radio frequency to rearrange the body's electromagnetic properties (see Figure 3-5). This scan is noninvasive and gives very detailed images with which to diagnose and follow pathological change.

The Extraocular Muscles

The bulbar fascia, or Tenon's capsule, is the connective tissue that surrounds the globe from the limbus and extends posteriorly to the optic nerve. It is dense and elastic, allowing the globe to move smoothly. Fat acts as a cushion between Tenon's capsule and the bony orbit, to absorb any pressure to the eyeball. Fat within the muscle cone serves to protect the optic nerve, surrounding blood vessels, and smaller nerves.

The six extraocular muscles (EOMs, Figure 5-7) move the eyes into the different positions of gaze. They are the superior rectus, inferior rectus, medial rectus, lateral rectus, inferior oblique, and superior oblique. The four rectus muscles originate (attach to bone for structural support) at the apex of the bony orbit in a fibrous tissue ring called the annulus of Zinn (or the circle of Zinn). The superior oblique originates in the orbital apex but is not part of the annulus of Zinn. The inferior oblique originates at the anterior nasal orbital floor.

Between the muscles is a cobweb-like tissue known as the intermuscular septum, which acts as an adhesive connection between the muscles. This septum is also a part of the annulus of Zinn.

The EOMs connect to the globe by stiff tendons at sites called insertions. The four rectus muscles simply come forward and attach to the sclera behind the limbus: the superior rectus at 7.5 mm, the lateral rectus at 7 mm, the inferior rectus at 6.75 mm, and the medial rectus at 5.5 mm (Figure 5-8). This configuration is known as the spiral of Tillaux (pronounced teh-LOW). The inferior oblique passes over the inferior oblique and under the lateral rectus muscles to attach at a point 17 mm from the limbus. The superior oblique passes through a cartilage "loop" called the trochlea (which is attached to the frontal bone and acts as a pulley), and then under the superior rectus muscle and to the globe. Its insertion runs perpendicular to the limbus (rather than parallel to it, as do the other muscles) from 13.8 to 18.8 mm (thus the width of the tendon at insertion is 5 mm).

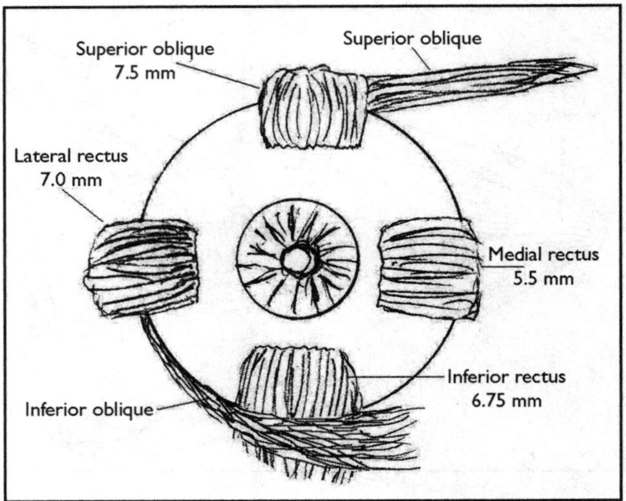

Figure 5-8. Schematic of the EOMs showing the distance each of the rectus muscles inserts from the limbus, creating the spiral of Tilleaux. (Adapted from a drawing by Holly Hess Smith. Gayton JL, Ledford JK. *The Crystal Clear Guide of Sight for Life*. Lancaster, PA: Starburst Publishers, 1996.)

Table 5-1
Muscle Measurements

Muscle	Length	Limbus to Insertion	Muscle Plane Angle
Superior rectus	42 mm	7.5 mm	23 degrees
Inferior rectus	40 mm	6.75 mm	23 degrees
Medial rectus	41 mm	5.5 mm	0 degrees
Lateral rectus	40.5 mm	7.0 mm	0 degrees
Superior oblique	59.5 mm*	13.8 to 18.8 mm	54 degrees
Inferior oblique	37 mm	17 mm	51 degrees

*SO total length, 19.5 mm of it is tendon

Adapted from Hansen VC. A Systematic Approach to Strabismus. *Thorofare, NJ: SLACK Incorporated; 1998.*

Anatomy (Table 5-1)

Superior Rectus (SR)

Origin: Crosses anterolaterally from the upper part of the annulus tendon, superolaterally to the optic foramen and sheath of the optic nerve, and attaches to the sclera 7.5 mm from the cornea by a 5.8-mm tendon

Muscle plane angle: 23 degrees

Size: 42 mm in length and 9 mm wide

Innervation: Superior division of the third cranial nerve (CN III/oculomotor nerve)

Blood supply: Lateral muscular branch of the ophthalmic arteries

Actions: Primary action—elevation; secondary action—intorsion; tertiary action—adduction

Inferior Rectus (IR)

Origin: Attaches below the optic foramen, passes forward anterolaterally along the floor of the orbit, and attaches to the sclera 6.75 mm from the cornea by a 5.5 mm tendon

Muscle plane angle: 23 degrees

Size: 40 mm long and 9 mm wide (the shortest of the recti muscles)

Innervation: Branch of the inferior division of the third cranial nerve (CN III/oculomotor) nerve)

Blood supply: Medial muscular branch of the ophthalmic artery

Actions: Primary action—depression; secondary action—extorsion; tertiary action—adduction

Medial Rectus (MR)

Origin: It has a wide attachment to the medial and inferior part of the optic foramen, then passes along the medial wall or the orbit, and inserts into the sclera 5.5 mm from the cornea by a 3.7-mm tendon

Muscle plane angle: 0 degrees

Size: 41 mm long (the largest and strongest EOM)

Innervation: Branch from the inferior division of the third cranial nerve (CN III/oculomotor)

Blood supply: Medial muscular branch of the ophthalmic artery

Action: Adduction

Lateral Rectus (LR)

Origin: Attaches to both parts of the annulus tendon (where they cross at the superior orbital fissure), passes forward along the lateral orbital wall, and attaches at the sclera 7.0 mm from the cornea by an 8.8-mm tendon

Muscle plane angle: 0 degrees

Size: 40.5 mm long

Innervation: Sixth cranial nerve (CN VI/abducens nerve)

Blood supply: Lacrimal artery and lateral muscular branch of the ophthalmic arteries

Action: Abduction

Note: Beginning superiorly on the right globe with the SR and moving around the eye counterclockwise, notice that the insertion-to-limbus distances of the muscle insertions decrease: the SR is 7.7 mm, the LR 7.0 mm, the IR 6.5 mm, and the MR 5.5 mm. The pattern produced by this steady change is known as the spiral of Tillaux.

Superior Oblique (SO)

Origin: Attaches superior medially to the optic foramen by a narrow tendon, passes forward between the orbital roof through the trochlea (a loop of cartilage on the frontal bone), turns back to the posterior part of the globe, and inserts inferior to the superior rectus in a fan-like, wide insertion; the 5-mm insertion runs 13.8 to 18.8 mm from the limbus

Muscle plane angle: 54 degrees

Size: Attachment 40 mm long to trochlea, then 19.5 mm of tendon to insertion (the longest, thinnest EOM)

Blood supply: Lateral or upper muscular branch of the ophthalmic artery

Innervation: Fourth cranial nerve (CN IV/trochlear nerve)

Actions: Primary action—intorsion; secondary action—depression; tertiary action—abduction

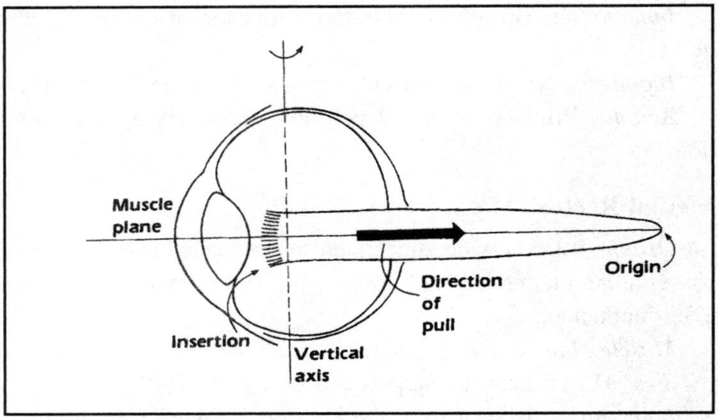

Figure 5-9. Muscle plane of the medial rectus. (Reprinted with permission from Hansen VC. *A Systematic Approach to Strabismus.* Thorofare, NJ: SLACK Incorporated; 1998.)

Inferior Oblique (IO)

Origin: From the anterior nasal orbital floor, it passes back to the nasal orbital wall and arcs laterally, then runs posterior around the globe, and inserts under the lateral rectus anterior to the trochlear area; the insertion is 17 mm from the limbus

Muscle plane angle: 51 degrees

Size: 37 mm long

Blood supply: Median or inferior branch of the supraorbital artery

Innervation: Third cranial nerve (CN III/oculomotor nerve)

Actions: Primary action—extorsion; secondary action—elevation; tertiary action—abduction

Physiology

The ability to look in different directions is made possible by the various origin and insertion sites of the muscles in relation to each other and to the center of the globe (Figures 5-9 through 5-12). The EOMs undergo simultaneous relaxation and contraction to move the eyes in tandem and are coordinated by specific nerves (see previous section). The "rules" that govern ocular movement are as follows:

- Sherington's law of reciprocal innervation—In the same eye, when one muscle contracts, the opposite (antagonist) muscle relaxes.
- Hering's law of equal innervation—When an impulse is sent to an EOM of one eye, the corresponding (yoke) muscle in the other eye is also stimulated to perform the same action.

Ocular movements are also partially controlled by fusion, or the ability of the eyes to lock onto an object, enabling them to align in order to keep the object image on each fovea. The fused image helps bond the eyes into coordinated movements.

The subject of ocular motility is a complex one; for a detailed discussion please see the Basic Bookshelf title *A Systematic Approach to Strabismus*. For the purposes of this text, here are some basic terms regarding ocular movements.

- vergence: Simultaneous ocular movement in which the eyes move away from or toward one another
  - ❖ convergence: Both eyes move inward toward the nose (as when looking at a near object)

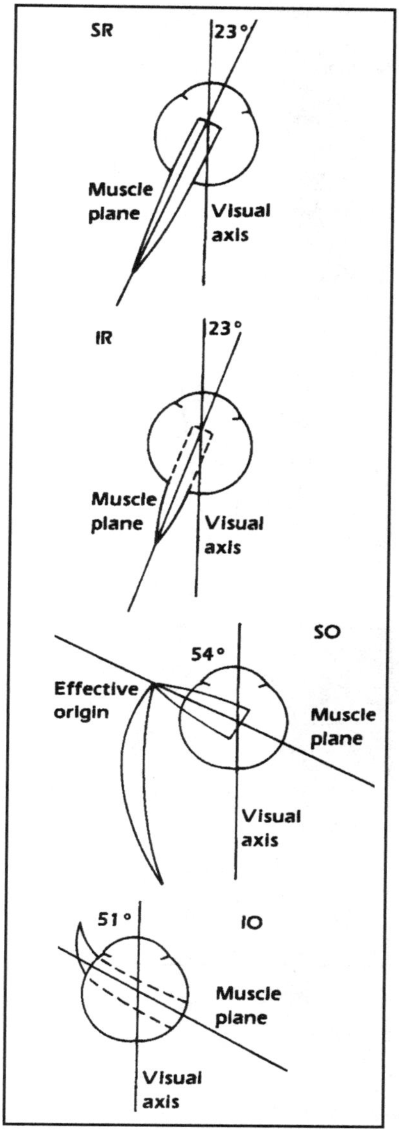

Figure 5-10. Muscle planes of the cyclovertical muscles. (Reprinted with permission from Hansen VC. *A Systematic Approach to Strabismus.* Thorofare, NJ: SLACK Incorporated; 1998.)

- divergence: Both eyes move outward, away from the nose (as when looking from a near object to a distant object)

- duction: Movement of a single eye from one position to another
  - abduction: Eye moves laterally (ie, away from the nose and toward the ear)
  - adduction: Eye moves medially (ie, toward the nose)
  - cycloduction: Rotation of the eye around its visual axis, as when the head is tilted
    - excycloduction: Rotation of the eye away from the nose (right eye when head is tilted toward the left; left eye when head is tilted to the right)
    - incycloduction: Rotation of the eye toward the nose (right eye when head is tilted toward the right; left eye when head is tilted to the left)

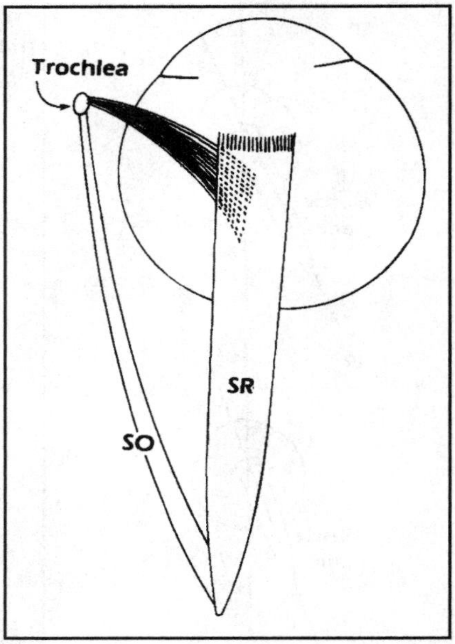

Figure 5-11. Superior oblique as related to superior rectus, right eye. (Reprinted with permission from Hansen VC. *A Systematic Approach to Strabismus.* Thorofare, NJ: SLACK Incorporated; 1998.)

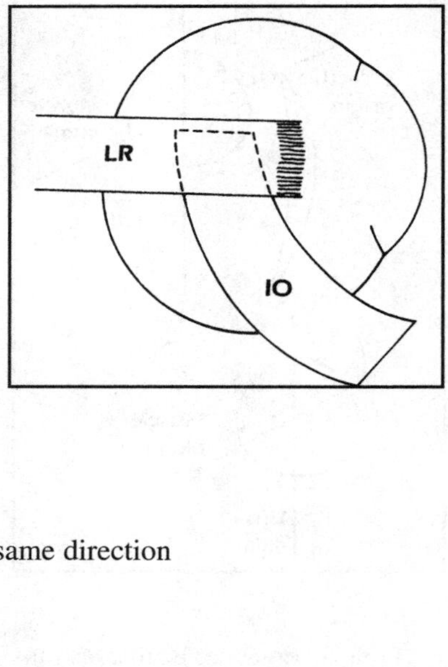

Figure 5-12. Inferior oblique as related to lateral rectus, right eye. (Reprinted with permission from Hansen VC. *A Systematic Approach to Strabismus.* Thorofare, NJ: SLACK Incorporated; 1998.)

- ❖ infraduction: Eye moves into downgaze
- ❖ supraduction: Eye moves into upgaze

- version: Simultaneous movement of both eyes in the same direction
  - ❖ dextroversion: Both eyes move to the right
  - ❖ infraversion: Both eyes move down
  - ❖ levoversion: Both eyes move to the left
  - ❖ supraversion: Both eyes move up

Evaluation of the Extraocular Muscles

Several simple motility tests evaluate the function of the EOMs. The *range of motion (ROM)* test evaluates the actions of each of the EOMs by having the patient voluntarily move the eyes into various positions (Figure 5-13). The *cross-cover test* is used to determine the presence or absence of a strabismus, as well as its direction. Once detected, the *cover-uncover test* can be used to determine if the strabismus is constant (tropia) or latent (phoria). *Prism testing* is used to measure the amount of phoria or tropia present. Various *stereo tests* can be employed to detect

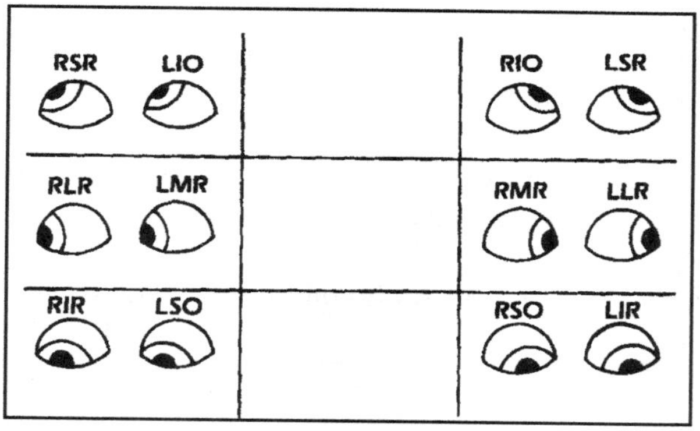

Figure 5-13. Diagnostic directions of gaze. (Reprinted with permission from Hansen VC. *A Systematic Approach to Strabismus*. Thorofare, NJ: SLACK Incorporated; 1998.)

and measure the patient's ability to fuse. These tests are all described in detail in the Basic Bookshelf titles *Clinical Skills for the Ophthalmic Examination: Basic Procedures* and *A Systematic Approach to Strabismus*.

Forced duction is a test to evaluate the potential physical movement of an eye with restricted movement. Under topical anesthetic, forceps are used to attempt to forcibly move the eye into the positions of restricted movement.

Electronystagmography (ENG) measures eye movements via electrodes and a computer as the patient tracks objects side-to-side. Often the tracking movements are stimulated by an optokinetic drum, a vertical rotating cylinder with vertical alternating black and white stripes, which is spun. The movement of the eyes is similar to watching passing fence posts when riding in a car. ENG can also be used to evaluate nystagmus.

Electromyography (EMG) is used to evaluate individual EOM function. After a drop of topical anesthetic is instilled, a thin needle (attached to a computer) is inserted into the muscle being tested. A normal muscle will create a "blip" (video) and a "chirp" (audio). A paralyzed muscle will cause no audio or video response. A weak muscle will cause a weaker response than that of a normally functioning muscle.

Glossary of Common Disorders

endophthalmitis*: Inflammation of the internal ocular tissues, occasionally an infection after surgery or penetrating injury, that can lead to loss of vision and of the eye itself if not controlled.

esophoria: Latent strabismus in which the nonfixating eye turns inward when fusion is disrupted.

esotropia: Strabismus in which the nonfixating eye turns inward.

exophoria: Latent strabismus in which the nonfixating eye turns outward when fusion is disrupted.

exophthalmos (also called proptosis): Condition in which the globe protrudes abnormally.

exotropia: Strabismus in which the nonfixating eye turns outward.

hypertropia: Strabismus in which the nonfixating eye turns upward.

hypotropia: Strabismus in which the nonfixating eye turns downward.

nystagmus*: Rapid, rhythmic, involuntary eye movements; nystagmus is classified according to the direction of the motion (horizontal is most common) and the stimuli that cause it to occur.

phoria: Strabismus that is evident only when fusion is disrupted.

strabismus: A misalignment of the eyes; an eye may be turned inward, outward, upward, or downward; the misalignment may be constant (tropia), intermittent, or latent (phoria; only evident when fusion is disrupted).

sympathetic ophthalmia*: Condition in which trauma or intraocular foreign body leading to uveitis in one eye is followed by uveitis in the other uninjured eye a few weeks later; in rare cases, it causes a loss of sight in both eyes.

tropia: Strabismus that is present either constantly or intermittently without fusion disruption.

* These definitions are used with permission from Ledford JK, Hoffman J. *Quick reference dictionary of eyecare terminology, fifth edition.* Thorofare, NJ: SLACK Incorporated; 2008.

CHAPTER 6

Conjunctiva, Episclera, and Sclera

Sheila Coyne Nemeth, COMT
Carolyn Shea, COMT

KEY POINTS

- The conjunctiva is the vascular mucous membrane that covers the anterior globe and the inner surface of the eyelids. This membrane plays a role in the immunological defense system of the external eye.
- The bulbar conjunctiva covers the globe itself, while the palpebral conjunctiva is attached to the tarsal plates of the eyelids.
- The episclera is the outermost layer of the sclera and has an extensive blood supply from the anterior ciliary arteries. Inflammation makes these vessels much more visible (when viewed with a slit lamp), as they lie just posterior to the bulbar conjunctiva.
- The sclera is the firm, protective, white housing for the inner contents of the globe. It is composed of dense collagen fibers.

Conjunctiva

The conjunctiva is the vascular mucous membrane that covers the anterior globe and the inner surface of the eyelids (Figure 6-1). ("Conjunctiva" is probably from the Latin *conjugation*, meaning joining together or blending.) The upper and lower pockets formed by the reflection of the conjunctiva onto the globe from the inner surface of the lids are known as the superior and inferior fornices.

In the body, mucous membranes line structures that open directly to exterior surfaces. The epithelial layer of any mucous membrane, including the conjunctiva, secretes mucus. Mucus is an excellent lubricant. It may also contain infection-fighting cells. Thus, the conjunctiva plays a role in the immunological defense system of the external eye and produces the mucus that is critically needed for tear film stability. Without the mucin layer of the tear film, the other tear layers destabilize, and the cornea can become compromised by exposure, drying, malnutrition, or infection. Mucus also lubricates the globe to reduce friction and adhesion of the lids.

Disorders that cause a decrease in the number of the conjunctiva's mucin-producing goblet cells are accompanied by conjunctival xerosis (drying). This drying is followed by keratinization, where the normally moist mucous membrane is replaced by an epithelium that is similar to skin. There may be increased mucus production in disorders such as keratoconjunctivitis sicca (KCS). The mucin strands frequently seen in KCS may be due to a change in the ratio of mucus to oil and water in these patients.

Because of its external position, the conjunctiva is subject to infection, foreign bodies, chemical splashes, etc. The typical conjunctival reaction to such occurrences is redness (hyperemia), swelling (chemosis), and exudation (mucus, tears, or pus).

Bulbar Conjunctiva

The conjunctiva is classified according to its location (Figure 6-2). The bulbar conjunctiva covers the globe itself. It is loosely attached, and moves when pushed with a cotton-tipped applicator. The conjunctiva is normally transparent with subtle vessels coursing through it, unless it becomes irritated. (Classically, any redness of the bulbar conjunctiva has been incorrectly referred to as "pink eye," a lay term for conjunctivitis.

The superficial bulbar conjunctival epithelium is continuous with the corneal epithelium. When the corneal epithelium is débrided, it may be resurfaced by limbal conjunctival epithelial cells "sliding" over.

The looseness of the bulbar conjunctiva makes it ideal for the creation of filtering blebs. These are surgically created pockets designed to allow aqueous to drain from the anterior chamber—lowering the intraocular pressure (IOP) in glaucoma.

Palpebral Conjunctiva

The *palpebral* (Latin for "eyelids") conjunctiva is firmly attached to the tarsal plate of the eyelids. One must pull the lower lid down or evert the upper lid to view the palpebral conjunctiva (Figure 6-3).

Two common pathologic changes that occur in this conjunctival surface are follicles and papillae. Follicles are clear mounds more common to the lower lid and are significant of an ocular irritant, allergic response, or viral lymphocytic reaction. Papillae (Latin for "little mounds") are fine, hyperemic elevations more common to the upper lid. They are associated with inflammation and infection.

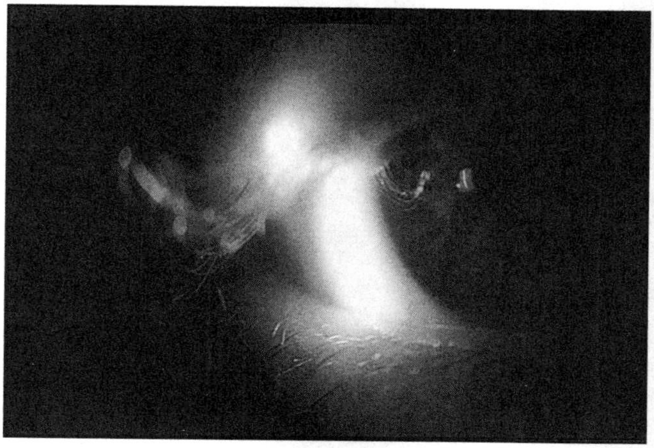

Figure 6-1. Slit lamp view of conjunctiva, episclera, and sclera. (Photo by Val Sanders. Reprinted with permission from Ledford JK, Sanders VN. *The Slit Lamp Primer, Second Edition.* Thorofare, NJ: SLACK Incorporated; 2006.)

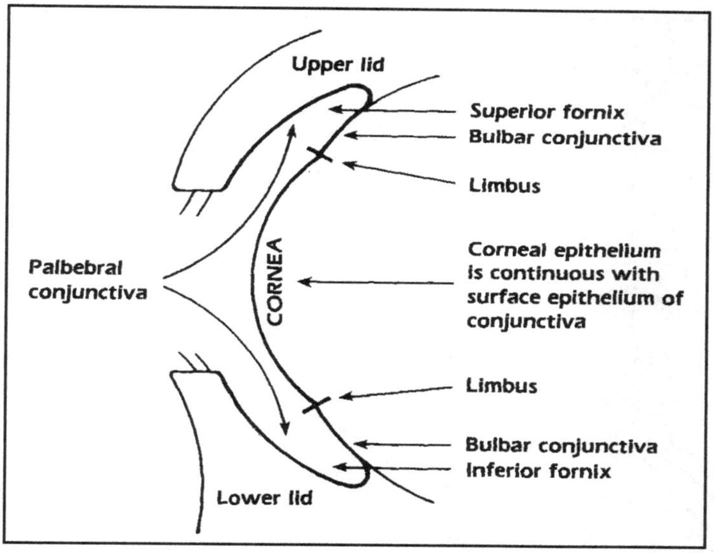

Figure 6-2. Cross-section of conjunctival topography. (Reprinted with permission from Nemeth SC, Shea CA. *Medical Sciences for the Ophthalmic Assistant.* Thorofare, NJ: SLACK Incorporated; 1988.)

Episclera

The episclera is the outermost layer of the sclera. It is loose connective tissue and anatomically merges with the underlying scleral stroma. The episclera has an extensive blood supply from the anterior ciliary arteries. These blood vessels are posterior to the bulbar conjunctiva and are usually only visible to the examiner when there is inflammation of the episclera (episcleritis).

The episclera is continuous with Tenon's capsule, the tissue encasing each EOM. The episclera also acts as a synovial membrane (like that which lines joints) to enable smooth eye movements.

Sclera

In lay terms, the sclera is the "white of the eye" (Figure 6-4). The function of the sclera is to provide a firm protective coat for the intraocular contents. The sclera is composed of dense

Figure 6-3. Palpebral conjunctiva.

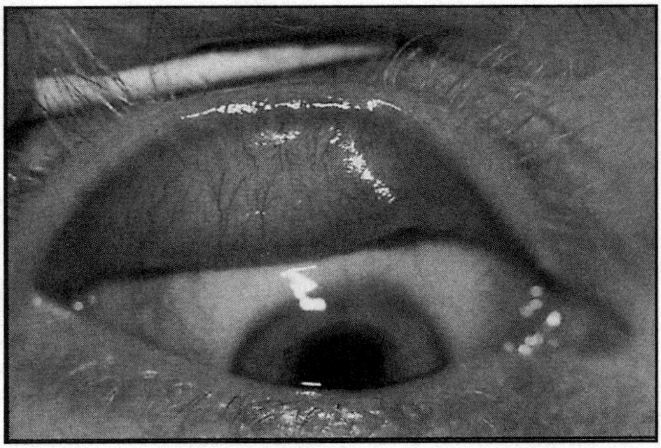

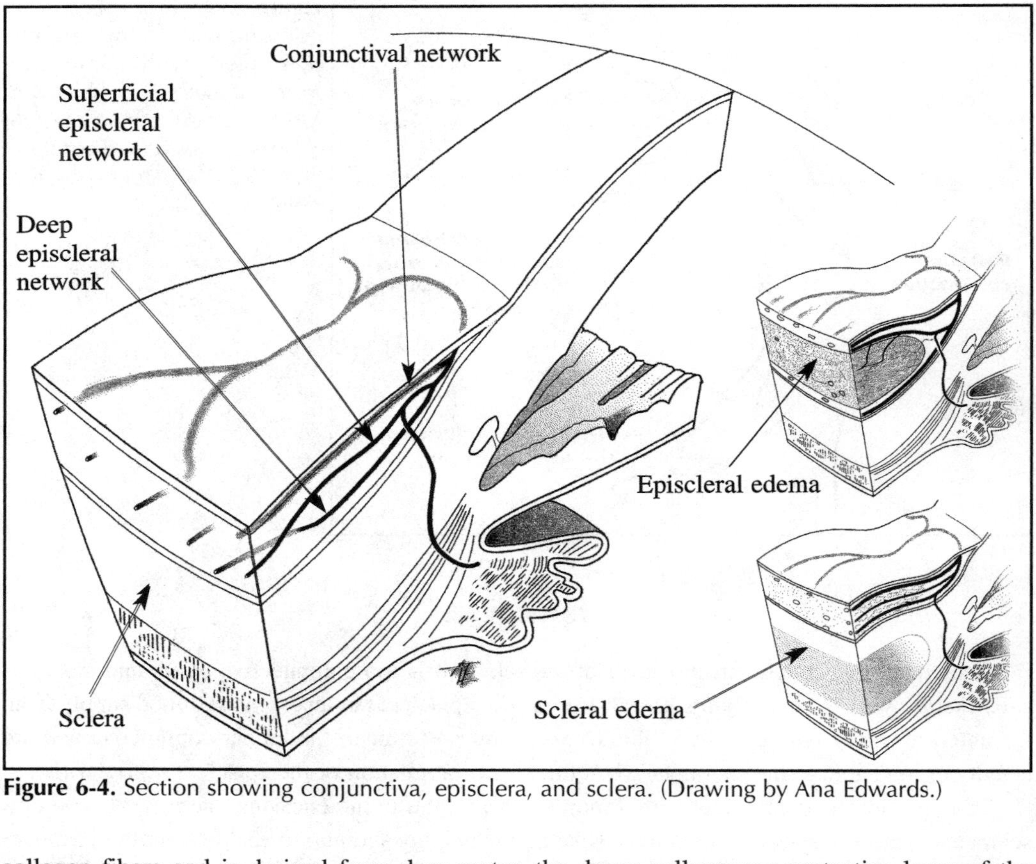

Figure 6-4. Section showing conjunctiva, episclera, and sclera. (Drawing by Ana Edwards.)

collagen fibers and is derived from dura mater, the dense collagenous protective layer of the brain. Normally the sclera is white, perhaps with a few pigmented spots, depending on the general pigmentation of the individual. In darker races, a collection of pigment is often found at the exit site of the anterior ciliary arteries. This can be confused with malignant changes.

The sclera is composed of collagen fibers arranged in a haphazard network. It is interesting to note that the cornea is composed of the same type of fibers. However, the corneal fibers are arranged in a lattice pattern, making the tissue transparent. Another factor that contributes to the differences between the cornea and sclera is that the cornea is dehydrated. The corneal endothelium acts as a pump to keep fluid out of the tissue, retaining the cornea's clarity. The scleral tissue, on the other hand, is opaque because it is hydrated.

The sclera is an elastic tissue, and this elasticity (referred to as scleral rigidity) can be a factor when measuring IOP by indentation methods, such as the Schiøtz tonometer. If the sclera is unusually distendable, the weight of the tonometer will cause the sclera to expand. This creates a falsely low IOP reading. Scleral rigidity is not considered to be a problem in applanation tonometry.

Jaundice can cause a yellowish scleral discoloration due to elevated bile levels. Yellowing can also occur with fatty deposits associated with aging. Certain connective tissue disorders can cause a bluish appearance due to scleral thinning and subsequent increased visibility of the deeper choroidal tissue. The sclera may also be thinner (and bluer) in childhood.

The sclera is continuous with a sieve-like network called the lamina cribrosa. The optic nerve exits the eye through this network. The long and short posterior ciliary nerves pierce the sclera anteriorly. The sclera is avascular and depends on the episclera for its vascular nutrition.

Since the sclera is composed primarily of collagen, it suffers from the destructive processes of the autoimmune diseases that affect systemic collagen. Collagen diseases include rheumatoid arthritis, sarcoidosis, and lupus.

The sclera is constantly being subjected to IOP and external environmental pressure changes. In certain diseases, such as congenital glaucoma, the sclera may be stretched, or ectatic.

Evaluation of Conjunctiva, Episclera, and Sclera

If *epinephrine drops* are instilled into a red eye, the blood vessels of the bulbar conjunctiva will constrict, making the eye whiter. The deeper episcleral vessels do not bleach with epinephrine use. This fact can be used as a diagnostic aid in assessing ocular injection.

The conjunctiva may be examined with a *penlight* and the naked eye but is better evaluated under the *slit lamp microscope*. A normal bulbar conjunctiva is essentially clear and moveable. A healthy palpebral conjunctiva is smooth and pink.

The *slit lamp examination* of the episclera and sclera is often aimed at evaluating inflammation of these tissues. It is important to ascertain the depth of inflammation and which vessels are being affected. Determination of scleral edema is the critical issue, as episcleritis does not involve the sclera. Some of the most useful illumination techniques are listed below. (For a complete guide to slit lamp use, see the Basic Bookshelf title *The Slit Lamp Primer, Second Edition.*)

- Diffuse illumination helps identify the particular configuration of the vessels involved. In episcleritis, the congested vessels are in a radial pattern, while scleritis may involve new, abnormal vessel formation around avascular areas.
- Slit beam illumination (optic section) utilizing the narrow optical section can assist in detecting the depth of vascular engorgement and scleral edema. In episcleritis, the anterior slit lamp beam is bowed forward from the episcleral edema, while the posterior slit lamp beam is flat (against normal sclera). With the underlying scleral edema of scleritis, this posterior slit lamp beam is bowed forward from the abnormal tissue inflammation.
- Viewing the episclera and sclera with a *green filter* ("red-free") will cause red vessels to appear darker and blacker, giving more contrast to subtle red vessels. This helps the examiner differentiate areas of dominant vascular congestion and other areas that are avascular.

Glossary of Common Disorders

chemosis: Swelling or edema of the bulbar conjunctiva.

conjunctivitis: Inflammation of the conjunctiva, which can be caused by bacteria, viruses, or allergens. Symptoms can include redness ("pink eye"), irritation (grittiness), swelling, discharge (exudates), and photophobia (sensitivity to light).

episcleritis: Inflammation of the episclera; on slit lamp exam, the inflamed vessels are often in a radial pattern.

exudation: Accumulation of by-products produced by the inflammatory process of the body. The discharge can be clear or mucoid or can cause the eyelids to "stick together" as in a viral or bacterial infection.

follicles: Clear, oval mounds on the palpebral conjunctival surface (most frequently the lower lid surface) that indicate ocular irritant, allergic response, or viral lymphocytic reaction.

hyperemia: Literally, "too much redness from blood." Clinically, the term *injection* is used for documenting the degree of redness observed on exam.

keratoconjunctivitis sicca: Inflammation of the cornea and conjunctiva often associated with dry eye.

papillae: Fine, hyperemic elevations most common to the palpebral conjunctival surface of the upper lid and associated with inflammation and infection.

scleritis: inflammation of the sclera; patients with diseases affecting the collagen system of the body (ie, rheumatoid arthritis and systemic lupus erythematosus) are especially prone.

subconjunctival hemorrhage (SCH): Bleeding occurring beneath the bulbar conjunctival membrane; frequently occur after heavy lifting, sneezing, or constant coughing. It is self-limiting and self-absorbing; there is minimal or no pain/discomfort.

xerosis: Drying of a mucous membrane, in this case the conjunctiva, due to a decrease in the goblet cells, which produce lubricating mucin.

Chapter 7

The Cornea

Tammy Langley, COT

Janice K. Ledford, COMT

KEY POINTS

- The cornea is the strongest refractive entity within our visual system, contributing two-thirds of the refractive power of the eye.
- The cornea is made up of five layers—epithelium, Bowman's membrane, stroma, Descemet's membrane, and endothelium.
- The corneal epithelium is one of the fastest healing tissues of the body.
- The stroma makes up 90% of the cornea's structure.
- The corneal endothelium functions as a water pump to maintain proper tissue hydration.
- The anatomy and physiology of the cornea are both geared toward one end—corneal clarity.

If there really is a window to the soul, then it is the cornea. This remarkable tissue, representing one-sixth of the external globe, is truly a work of art. When in top working order, the cornea is crystal clear. This provides a pristine medium through which to see (Figure 7-1). With its five layers (assisted by the tear film—see Chapter 4), it is the strongest refractive entity in our visual system, contributing two-thirds of the refractive power of the eye.

The optical power of the cornea equals approximately 42.0 to 43.0 diopters. (The average eye's total dioptric power is 57 to 62.) This refractive characteristic has spawned surgical procedures in which the cornea's shape is altered to change the refractive status of the eye. These include laser in situ keratomileusis (LASIK), laser epithelial keratomileusis (LASEK), laser photorefractive keratectomy, and others. (See the Basic Bookshelf title *Refractive Surgery for Eyecare Paraprofessionals*.)

The cornea's average diameter is about 11.7 mm across and 10.6 mm vertically. The cornea of the female tends to be about 0.1 mm smaller than that of the male. The cornea is thicker where it joins the limbus (1.1 mm) and thinner in the center (5.3 mm).

The central 4 mm of the cornea is the optic zone or corneal cap. The optic zone directly overlies the pupil and represents the portion of the cornea through which we have central vision. If the corneal cap is not spherical (ie, is curved more in one direction than another), then the condition of astigmatism exists (see Chapter 16). The anterior and posterior surfaces of the cornea are nearly parallel in the optic zone. However, the tissue thickens as it continues peripherally, so the anterior and posterior surfaces do not remain parallel but spread apart.

The average radius of the curvature of the cornea's anterior surface is 7.8 mm (range is 6.8 to 8.5 mm). The cornea's curvature changes, gradually becoming flatter as it approaches the limbus. Since the rest of the globe has a larger radius of curvature (averaging 11.5 mm), there is a slight groove at the limbus where the cornea and sclera meet.

The cornea's nerve supply comes from the ophthalmic branch of the trigeminal nerve (see Chapter 11). This enters the tissue mainly through the sclera via the long posterior ciliary nerves. A few enter via the episclera. After penetrating 2 to 3 mm into the cornea at the limbus, the nerves no longer have a myelin sheath. By the time the nerve endings reach the central cornea, they are faint, hair-like strands. This is an important feature in the clarity of the cornea.

The blood supply to the cornea comes via vessels in the conjunctiva, episclera, and sclera. Tiny capillaries barely cross the limbus into the corneal tissue, then loop back to the limbus. Thus, the normal cornea is largely an avascular tissue, another feature that contributes to corneal clarity. Most of the cornea's required oxygen comes from the atmosphere via the tear film (see Chapter 4).

The cornea is dehydrated tissue except for its internal and external surfaces. It is interesting to note that the corneal fibrils (made up of collagen) are essentially the same as those present in the sclera. The sclera, however, is a hydrated tissue. If the cornea becomes hydrated, it becomes opaque like the sclera. (Conversely, if the sclera becomes dehydrated, clear patches will appear.)

The cornea is made up of five layers (Figure 7-2). Each of these layers has a distinct function. From exterior to interior, the layers are (a) the epithelium, (b) Bowman's membrane, (c) the stroma (the substantia propria), (d) Descemet's membrane, and (e) the endothelium.

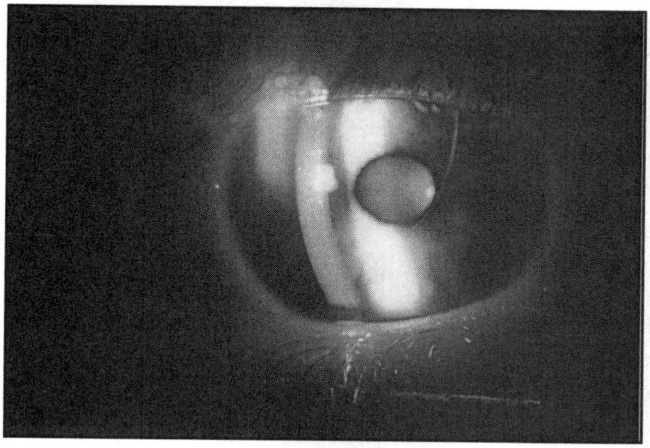

Figure 7-1. Slit lamp view of the cornea. (Photo by Val Sanders. Reprinted with permission from Ledford JK, Sanders VN. *The Slit Lamp Primer, Second Edition*. Thorofare, NJ: SLACK Incorporated; 2006.)

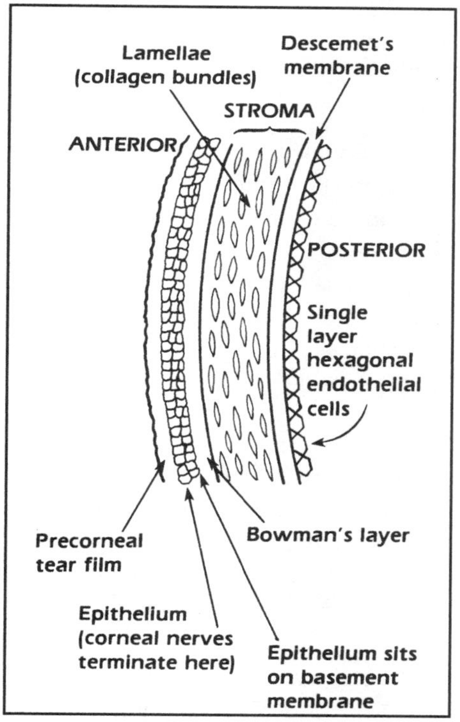

Figure 7-2. Histological cross-section of the cornea. (Reprinted with permission from Nemeth SC, Shea CA. *Medical Sciences for the Ophthalmic Assistant*. Thorofare, NJ: SLACK Incorporated; 1988.)

Anatomy

Epithelium

The epithelium is the outer-most layer of the cornea. It is bathed with tears during every blink, provides a smooth refractive surface, and protects the stroma from external injury.

Epithelial tissue is actually a continuation of the bulbar conjunctiva. The epithelium in the center of the cornea usually has five or six layers of cells. As the cornea thickens and moves out toward the limbus, as many as 10 layers or more can be found.

The epithelium has three forms of cells: two layers of flattened epithelial cells externally, followed by two or three layers of wing (polygonal) cells, and a single internal layer of basal cells (columnar in shape).

The basal cells are responsible for mitosis (reproduction of cells). The new cell begins as another basal cell then migrates upward, becoming a wing cell. Upward movement continues until the cell becomes an outer epithelial cell and is eventually shed. In addition, new epithelial basal cells migrate into the corneal epithelium from the limbus.

The external cell layer excretes a thin layer of mucin, which helps the epithelium bond with the mucin layer of the tear film. In addition, the outer-most cells have tiny projections (microvilli) that also play a role in the corneal/tear relationship.

The epithelium is nonpigmented, with the exception of darker races who can have some pigment in the periphery of the cornea. Running between the epithelial cells are the ends of sensory nerve fibers, which are very sensitive to pain. As these superficial cells age, they loose their attachment to each other and are flushed away with the tear film. They are replaced with new cells. (It is estimated that the entire epithelium is replaced every week.)

The epithelium is one of the fastest healing tissues of the body, regenerating in less than 24 hours. The epithelium heals without scarring; this is not true of some of the cornea's deeper layers.

Bowman's Membrane

Bowman's membrane is directly under the epithelium. It is acellular and made up of collagen fibers embedded in various intercellular substances. These fibrils are uniform in thickness and can measure 20 to 30 nm in diameter. They seem to be surrounded by mucoprotein. The anterior surface of Bowman's membrane is smooth, but the posterior surface is less defined as it merges into the stromal layer. Bowman's membrane acts as a barrier against micro-organisms, protecting the stroma. It cannot regenerate following trauma; if an injury extends into Bowman's membrane, a scar will result. Bowman's membrane ends abruptly at the limbus.

Stroma

The stroma is the most substantial layer of the cornea, comprising approximately 90% of the corneal tissue. It is made up of 200 to 250 transparent lamellae consisting of collagen fibrils in an extracellular matrix. The lamellae are laid down at right angles to each other (but do not interweave). This arrangement is very important because it contributes to the clarity of the cornea. (The sclera is made up of the same fibers, but they are arranged haphazardly, resulting in the sclera's opacity.)

Fibroblasts and keratocytes are also present throughout the stromal layer, lying between the lamellae. Fibroblasts (cells that can form collagen fibers) have long branching processes that reach in many directions from the cell body. The keratocytes (flattened stromal cells) have long extensions and are most often seen in the posterior stroma. Keratocytes assist in corneal healing by engulfing foreign particles.

The stroma also contains glycogen and small lipid droplets. Schwann cells (cells with a sheathing membrane) surround corneal nerves. Lymphocytes, macrophages, and on rare occasion, polymorphonuclear leukocytes may be present in the stroma as well. These cells play an important role when inflammation is present.

Descemet's Membrane

Descemet's membrane is at the posterior side of the stroma and is the basement membrane of the endothelium (innermost layer). It is composed of fine collagen fibers arranged in a hexagonal

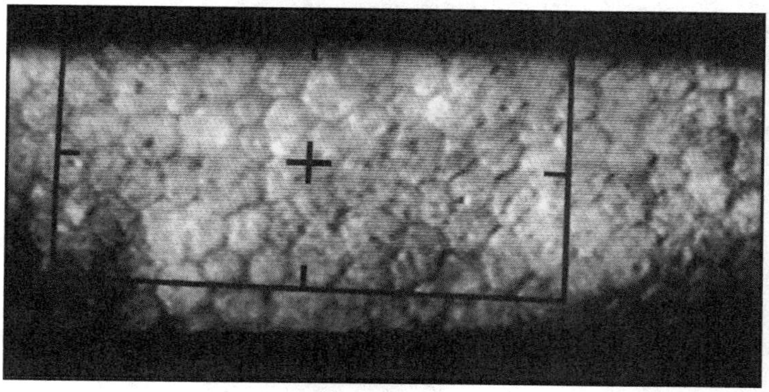

Figure 7-3. Corneal endothelium as seen with the specular microscope. (Photo by Val Sanders, COT, CRA.)

pattern and embedded in a matrix. This membrane is very thin at birth (3 mm) and thickens in adulthood to 12 mm.

There is a very clear delineation between the stroma and Descemet's membrane. Descemet's membrane provides a barrier to cells and vessels, protecting the more inferior portions of the eye. It can be easily separated from both the stroma and the endothelium.

Descemet's membrane overflows into the trabecula and ends at Schwalbe's ring (the line of Schwalbe). At the very periphery of the cornea there are minute protrusions of Descemet's membrane (that have some endothelium intermixed) into the anterior chamber. These protrusions are called Hassal-Henle bodies (or warts). Descemet's membrane can often be observed (through the slit lamp microscope) as curling up into the AC, especially in an aging eye or following significant corneal trauma.

Endothelium

The endothelium is a single layer of flattened cells that are polygonal in shape. The plasma membranes of the cells are interlocked, creating a honey-comb like appearance (Figure 7-3). Each cell has 20 to 30 tiny projections (microvilli) that protrude into the aqueous, providing an increased surface area for removing waste and obtaining nutrients.

An average of 500,000 cells make up this layer. However, the corneal endothelium does not have the ability to regenerate. With age, cells die and drop off. The remaining cells spread out and take up the space, preventing a break in the endothelium. In some cases, eventually the remaining cells can no longer cover the empty spaces, as in eye diseases like Fuchs' corneal dystrophy.

The corneal endothelium is a major contributor to the dehydrated state of the cornea. This layer acts as a water pump and is crucial in keeping fluid from entering into the corneal stroma. These "pumps" are located in each cell's lateral membrane and number around 3 million per cell.

Physiology

The clarity of the cornea is the product of its structure and physiology. Essential to this physiology is the endothelium's function as a barrier to the aqueous and as a pump to keep the stroma at the proper hydration. The tight junctures of the endothelial cells are paramount in both of these. Therefore, any decrease in cell numbers, or breaks between cells, can compromise the endothelium's ability to act as a barrier.

When everything is balanced properly, the stroma is about 75% hydrated. Further hydration results in edema, swelling, and loss of clarity. The process by which the endothelial pump works is complicated but includes levels of sodium, potassium, and enzymes, as well as osmotic pressure. To greatly simplify this system, one could say that the pump strives to maintain a situation in which the concentration of sodium is greater in the aqueous, so water would move from the stroma to the aqueous.

Endothelial compromise can occur in corneal dystrophies, in which cell loss plays a role. Another potential cause of cell loss is intraocular surgery, when the endothelium could be bumped (as with an intraocular lens [IOL] during cataract surgery). During angle-closure glaucoma, the increased IOP interferes with the pump mechanism, and corneal edema (one of the hallmarks of the disorder) occurs.

Oxygen for corneal metabolism (even for the endothelium) comes chiefly from the atmosphere. If the amount of oxygen available to the cornea is decreased, then corneal edema occurs. A measure of hypoxia (lack of oxygen) occurs naturally during sleep, when the eye is closed and less oxygen can get to the cornea. Essentially, everyone awakens with a small degree of edema. However, if hypoxia is protracted (as in the case of contact lens wear), corneal edema continues throughout the day. Neovascularization may also occur where new blood vessels grow into the corneal tissue in an attempt to provide the oxygen needed. Edema and neovascularization are the reasons that contact lens fitters pay such careful attention to the oxygen transmissibility of the various contact lens materials.

The corneal tissue has great tenacity when it comes to enduring injuries of many different types. The amount and the location of scarring varies almost as much as the many types of infections and injuries that are possible. If scarring occurs in the optic zone, vision will almost certainly be affected. Scarring that occurs in the periphery may not be noticed at all.

Evaluation of the Cornea

The *slit lamp biomicroscope* was designed with the cornea in mind. Because the microscope's light can be narrowed into a thin beam, evaluation of an optical section (thin slice) of the cornea is possible (Figure 7-4). Tangential illumination, specular reflection, and indirect illumination methods (proximal, sclerotic scatter, and retroillumination) can all be used for corneal evaluation.

Slit lamp examination of the corneal endothelium is further enhanced by the use of sodium fluorescein (NaFl). This yellow dye fluoresces when the cobalt blue filter of the slit lamp is used. Areas that take up stain (and glow under the blue light) represent areas where the epithelial surface has been broken.

Rose bengal is a stain that is used under the white light of the slit lamp. Areas of dead epithelium will stain pink with this dye.

Several other instruments are used to evaluate the cornea. The *pachymeter* is a contact instrument used to measure the cornea's thickness. This measurement is vital in planning refractive surgery as well as evaluating for glaucoma.

Specular microscopy is used to view the corneal endothelium (see Figure 7-3). This powerful microscope makes it possible to view the single layer of cells making up the endothelium. The picture is then evaluated for cell number and density. This test is sometimes used before intraocular surgery in order to discern whether or not the endothelium is healthy enough to withstand the trauma associated with the procedure. It is also used to follow patients with corneal endothelial dystrophy.

The *keratometer* is used to measure the curvature of the corneal cap. This information is used for refractometric purposes, IOL calculations, and contact lens fittings.

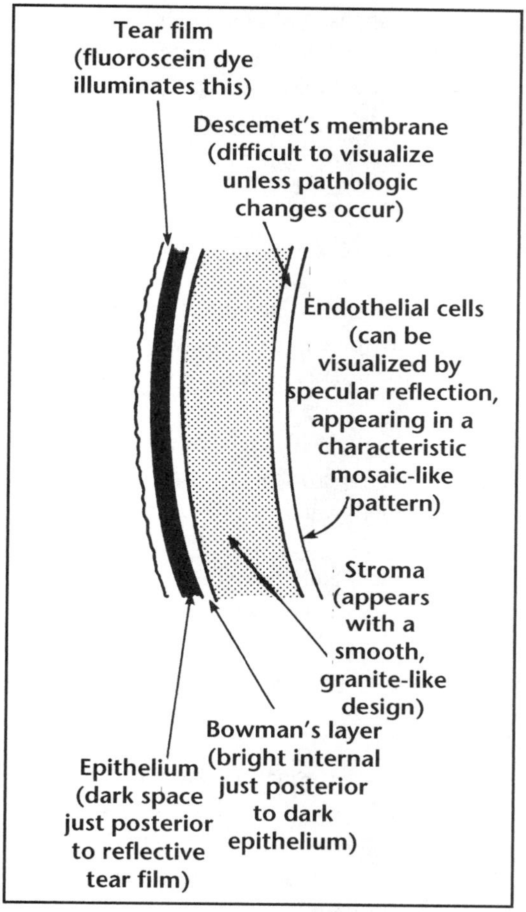

Figure 7-4. Optic section of the cornea as it appears under the slit lamp. (Reprinted with permission from Nemeth SC, Shea CA. *Medical Sciences for the Ophthalmic Assistant.* Thorofare, NJ: SLACK Incorporated; 1988.)

More sophisticated than keratometry is *corneal topography*, which provides a view of the curvature of the entire cornea. A computer generates a topographical map, which is largely used in refractive surgical planning. It is used to a lesser degree for difficult contact lens fits and to follow patients with keratoconus.

Placido's disk evaluates the cornea's reflection of a pattern of concentric rings. The examiner looks for the closeness of the rings to each other, as well as the shape of their curve, and notes these findings in the patient's chart. The disk provides information about the nature of the cornea's curvature, but no numerical measurements.

Confocal microscopy provides corneal imaging on a very minute (sometimes cellular) level. Its field of view is miniscule, and a wider view must be generated by scanning photography. The confocal microscope is used to identify pathogens (mainly nonbacterial in nature), evaluate postoperative refractive surgery problems, and assess healing. If a laser is used, the technique is called laser confocal microscopy.

Corneal thickness, as well as imaging the cornea (including LASIK flaps) can be done with *optical coherence tomography*. Another method of obtaining a three-dimensional corneal image is *B-scan ultrasound* if a 100-MHz probe is used.

The function of the cornea's sensory nerves can be evaluated by a *corneal sensitivity test*. This evaluation uses an instrument called an anesthesiometer. It involves gently touching the cornea with fine nylon filaments of varying lengths. The patient's response (or lack thereof) is noted in the chart, along with the length of the filament. (A simple yes/no evaluation of corneal sensitivity can be done by brushing the cornea with strands pulled from a cotton-tipped applicator.)

Evaluating corneal infections can be done via *cytology*, including Gram and Giemsa staining, and by *culturing* for bacteria, etc.

Glossary of Common Disorders/Conditions

abrasion*: Injury in which tissues are scraped from an area on the surface of the cornea, usually involving the corneal epithelium but possibly extending more deeply.

arcus: A creamy-colored ring (or partial ring) at the limbus, usually occurring with advancing age.

dystrophy*: General term for hereditary condition in which there is defective development or degeneration of corneal tissue (ie, Fuch's, lattice, map-dot-fingerprint).

edema: Hydration of the corneal tissues, which swell and cloud; usually indicates a malfunction in the endothelium.

guttata: General term referring to a spot or spots on the corneal endothelium.

infiltrates*: Whitish, cloudy particles in the cornea, often associated with infection or contact lens wear.

keratitis: General term for inflammation of the cornea; may be caused by bacteria, fungi, virus, exposure, injury, etc.

keratoconjunctivitis sicca: *See* definition on p. 54.

keratoconus* (also called ectatic corneal dystrophy): Progressive malformation of the cornea such that it is thin and cone-like in shape rather than rounded; causes painless visual distortion (due to astigmatism) and loss.

Krukenberg's spindles* (also called spindle cells): Small, round deposits of pigment on the corneal endothelium arranged in a central, vertical pattern; often associated with iritis, diabetes, and pigmentary glaucoma.

neovascularization: In the cornea, growth of abnormal blood vessels from the limbus into the normally vascular-free corneal tissues.

opacity: Any area on/in the cornea that is not transparent; the closer the opacity is to the optic axis, the more it will affect visual acuity.

pannus*: Condition in which blood vessels grow into the cornea, which then becomes fibrous and loses its transparency; may be classified according to type as allergic, glaucomatous, etc.

pterygium*: Triangular membrane of fleshy tissue extending from a base in the conjunctiva of the canthus toward and possibly onto the cornea; removed surgically if it begins to impinge on the optic axis.

ulcer: Condition in which there is tissue loss from the corneal surface, usually associated with infection (bacterial, fungal, or viral) but may also occur following chemical or physical trauma.

* These definitions are used with permission from Ledford JK, Hoffman J. *Quick reference dictionary of eyecare terminology, fifth edition.* Thorofare, NJ: SLACK Incorporated; 2008.

Chapter 8

Anterior and Posterior Chambers

Carolyn Shea, COMT

Sheila Coyne Nemeth, COMT

Mark DiSclafani, MD

R. Rand Allingham, MD

KEY POINTS

- The anterior segment is the small, asymmetric cavity of the globe that includes the lens and all structures anterior to the lens.
- The anterior segment is made up of the anterior chamber (AC) and posterior chamber (PC).
- The AC lies anterior to the iris (behind the cornea) and contains aqueous.
- The PC lies posterior to the iris and contains the lens.

The anterior segment of the eye is often identified simply as "the front of the eye." Now we will concentrate on the AC and PC, both part of the anterior segment. (The cornea is also a part of the AC, but was covered separately in Chapter 7.) An anterior segment surgeon is a surgeon who is trained in operations specific to glaucoma, cataracts, and cornea. Structures and entities in this chapter include the iris, pupil, ciliary body, aqueous, angle, and lens.

Evaluation of the Chambers

As a whole, the AC and PC can be evaluated via *ultrasound*. A-scan gives a one-dimensional view, valuable for measuring chamber depth and the location of structures. B-scan yields a two-dimensional evaluation of structures, often used to evaluate growths and foreign bodies. During surgery, the chambers may be visualized using endoscopy (scope-mounted camera).

Recently, new instruments have been developed that provide very high-resolution imaging of the anterior segment of the eye. One is *ultrasound biomicroscopy* (UBM), which provides high resolution (50 μm) by use of ultrasound transducers. The ultrasound probe is moved over the surface of the eye and records the anterior segment features (Figure 8-1). For example, angle-closure glaucoma due to pupillary block has been clearly demonstrated with this instrument.

In addition, a noncontact, stand-alone instrument called Visante (Carl Zeiss Meditec, Dublin, CA) has been introduced using high-resolution *optical coherence tomography* (OCT) for imaging the anterior segment of the eye. This device can measure corneal thickness as well as AC depth and AC angles. There is no need for ocular anesthesia or water bath with this instrument.

Evaluation of the specific AC structures are covered in the corresponding sections.

Iris and Pupil

The iris can be thought of as a colored muscular shutter attaching peripherally to the ciliary body. The central aperture, or opening, is the pupil. The primary function of the iris is to regulate the size of the pupil via the innervation of its muscles. The iris prevents excessive light from entering the system and helps to form clear images on the retina by preventing peripheral rays of light from entering the eye. The "f-stop" (aperture) of a camera is a simulation of the iris and pupil.

The pigmentation and surface topography of the iris vary from person to person (Figure 8-2A). Generally, brown irides appear to have an even, diffuse pigmentation throughout the iris surface and may have noticeable contraction furrows in the periphery. In diffuse lighting using a slit lamp, the surface view of blue irides appears to have more "hills and valleys" within the textured anterior surface. These valleys are iris crypts. There also may be scattered patches of deeper pigmentation, as well as iris freckles (nevi).

The stroma, or middle layer, is thickest at the pupil (Figure 8-2B). The stroma contains the dilator and sphincter muscles. These muscles affect the size of the pupil through the innervation of the autonomic (involuntary) nervous system (ANS). The dilator muscle, under sympathetic innervation of the ANS, runs radially in the stroma and functions to increase the amount of ambient light available to the retina. The sphincter muscle, on the other hand, is under parasympathetic innervation of the ANS and circles the pupillary border near the collarette. The sphincter serves to decrease the amount of light reaching the retina. Miosis is synonymous with constriction, the function of the sphincter muscle. Mydriasis is synonymous with dilation, the function of the dilator muscle. Pharmacologically, a miotic decreases and a mydriatic increases pupil diameter.

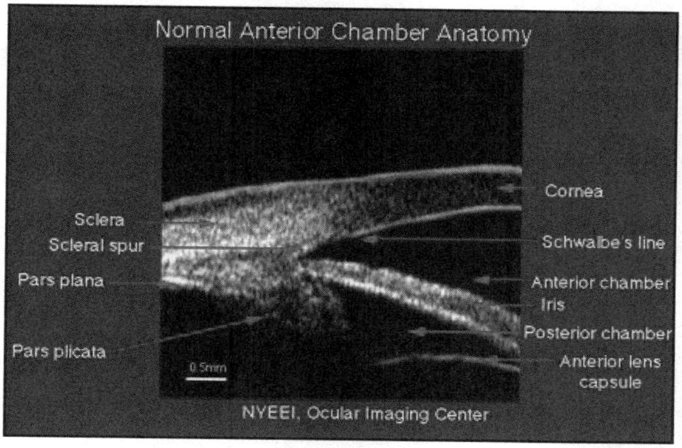

Figure 8-1. Ultrasound biomicroscopy image showing normal AC structures. (Photo courtesy of The Ocular Imaging Center/New York Eye and Ear Infirmary, New York, NY.)

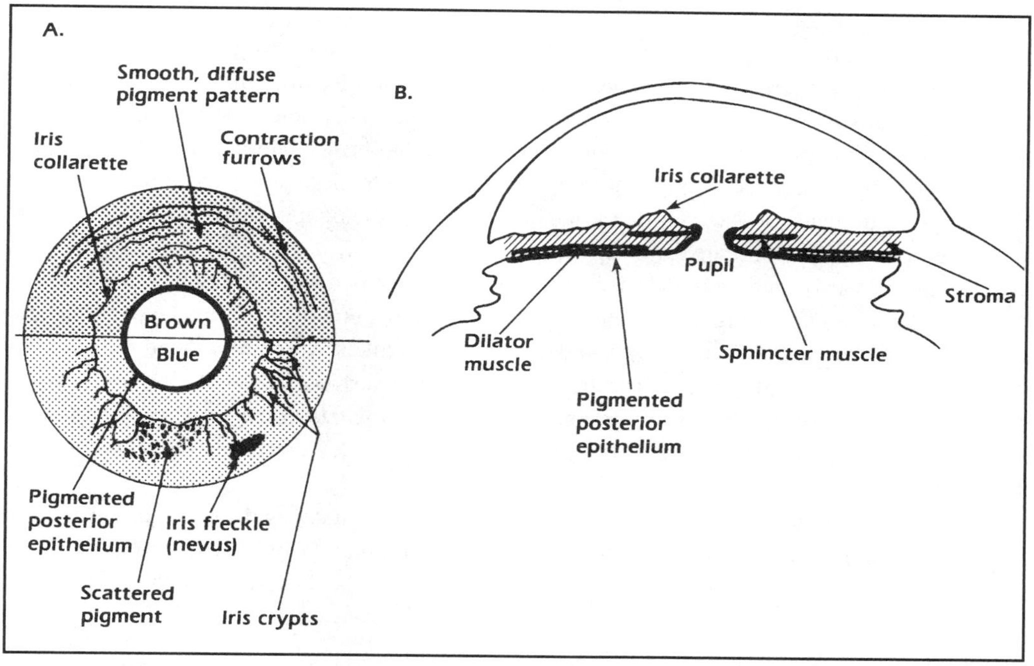

Figure 8-2. (A) External view of blue and brown irides. (B) Cross-section of iris anatomy. (Reprinted with permission from Nemeth SC, Shea CA. *Medical Sciences for the Ophthalmic Assistant.* Thorofare, NJ: SLACK Incorporated; 1988.)

The pupil is constantly adjusting in size due to the changing muscle tone of the dilator and sphincter muscles. These normal, small readjustments of the pupil are known as hippus. Normally the pupils are equal in size, but approximately one-quarter of the population has pupils of slightly different sizes (anisocoria).

The stroma also contains the pigment cells containing melanin, known as melanocytes, which constitute our genetically determined eye color. Brown eyes are genetically dominant to blue eyes. If both parents are blue-eyed, then the child will definitely have blue eyes. If one parent is brown-eyed and one parent is blue-eyed, then the chances are 50% (at the most) that the child will be blue-eyed.

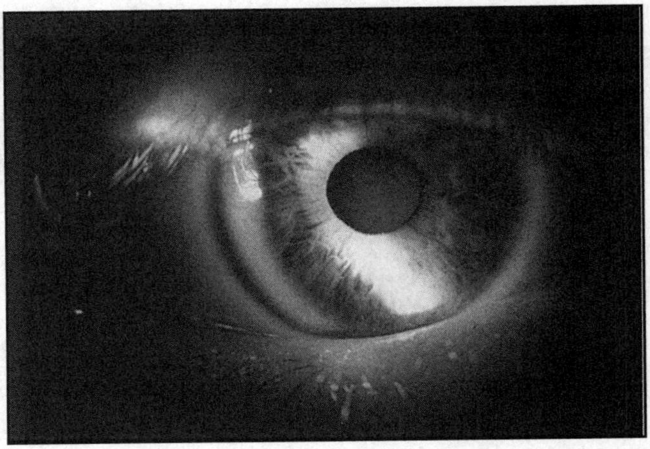

Figure 8-3. Slit lamp view of the iris and pupil. (Photo by Val Sanders. Reprinted with permission from Ledford JK, Sanders VN. *The Slit Lamp Primer, Second Edition*. Thorofare, NJ: SLACK Incorporated; 2006.)

People with less pigment in their system are often less tolerant of bright sunlight and glare. Pigment acts as an absorber of light; therefore, those without a lot of pigment are more photophobic (light sensitive). Consequently, you will find red-heads and blondes with blue eyes in the optical shops trying on sunglasses more often than those with brown hair and brown eyes. Albinism is a congenital absence of pigment in the pigmented epithelium as well as the stroma. The iris will transilluminate, or allow light to shine through, when the light is directed either obliquely from a point posterior to the limbus or directly through the pupil.

The most posterior surface of the iris is the posterior pigmented epithelium layer, which helps block peripheral light entering the system. Under the slit lamp, one may see this layer at the border of the pupil (the pupillary margin) as a darker frill of pigment wrapping around the margin.

Often thin, cobweb-like threads can be seen on the iris surface. These are pupillary membrane remnants. These thin threads represent embryologic remnants of the fetal vascular system that once served to nourish the anterior segment of the eye. They are most frequently seen in children.

The iris may be subject to tumors (both benign and malignant) and inflammation (iritis). Because the pupil is controlled by nerve impulses, any problem with these nerves may also produce an abnormality of function. (See Glossary of Common Disorders at the end of this chapter.)

Evaluation of the Iris and Pupil

The iris is best examined with the *slit lamp microscope* (Figure 8-3). The surface of the iris may be illuminated directly by shining the slit beam right onto the structure. The slit beam may also be shown through the pupil and allowed to reflect off the retina, illuminating the iris from behind (transillumination). This technique is ideal for evaluating the integrity of the iris (Figure 8-4). The slit lamp can also be used to examine the pupil's size and shape. *Slit lamp photography* may be used to create a permanent record of the pupil and iris.

Using a modified photo slit lamp, *fluorescein angiography* and *indocyanine green angiography* of the iris can be performed to evaluate the morphology and vascular dynamics of the anterior segment of the eye. It can clarify certain vascular abnormalities caused by systemic disease or local tumor-like lesions.

Pupillary reaction is usually tested with a penlight or muscle light. First, the light is shown into each eye individually (each pupil should constrict when the light hits either eye). Next, the

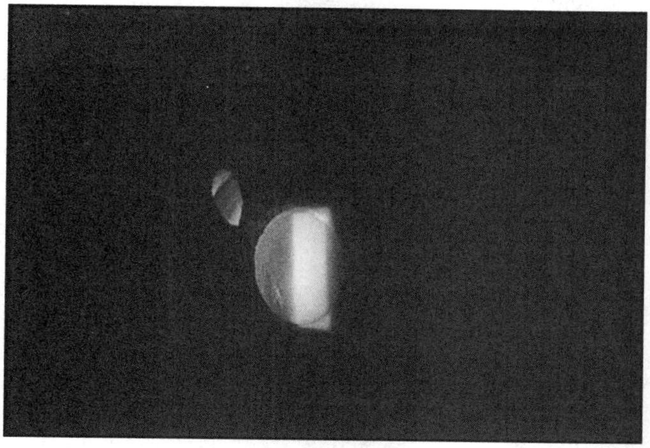

Figure 8-4. Iris transillumination showing iridotomy. (Photo by Val Sanders. Reprinted with permission from Ledford JK, Sanders VN. *The Slit Lamp Primer, Second Edition.* Thorofare, NJ: SLACK Incorporated; 2006.)

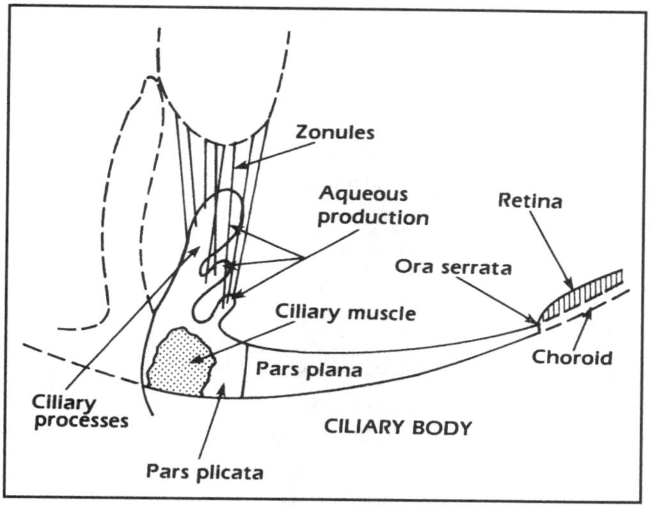

Figure 8-5. Ciliary body and related structures. (Reprinted with permission from Nemeth SC, Shea CA. *Medical Sciences for the Ophthalmic Assistant.* Thorofare, NJ: SLACK Incorporated; 1988.)

light is moved from one pupil to the other, comparing the reaction of one pupil with the other. Because pupil size and reaction are influenced by stimulation of the retina all the way back to the brain stem, pupil evaluation aids in the diagnosis of both ocular and nervous system disorders. How-to's and details of these techniques are given in the Basic Bookshelf title *Clinical Skills for the Ophthalmic Examination: Basic Procedures*.

The size of the pupil may be formally measured with a *pupillometer*. However, it is generally easier to compare the pupil to a template showing circles of various sizes (often printed on near vision cards). *Pupillography* uses infrared lighting to produce a photographic image of the undilated, dark-adapted pupil. (A normal flash would cause the pupil to constrict.) This technique often uses a video camera so that the response of the pupil to various lighting situations can be documented. Neither pupillometry or pupillography is in widespread use.

Ciliary Body

The ciliary body lies between the iris and the choroid (Figure 8-5). It contains pigment and a rich vascular network. It is divided into two sections, the anterior pars plicata and the more posterior pars plana. Chronic inflammation of the ciliary body may be called iridocyclitis (if anterior), pars planitis (if posterior), or uveitis (a nonlocalizing term).

Anatomy

The Pars Plicata

The pars plicata is comprised of two important structures, the ciliary muscle and the ciliary processes.

The ciliary muscle controls the ability to accommodate (change focus) at different distances. It does this by altering the shape of the lens. The lens and the ciliary muscle work together to allow us to see the fine needlepoint work we are doing and then instantaneously refocus in on the TV as we look across the room. (This will be covered in more detail in Chapter 15.)

The ciliary processes are small, finger-like projections located in the PC posterior to the iris. These processes serve as connecting sites for the lens zonules, anchoring the zonules to the ciliary muscle. The processes also produce aqueous humor, the fluid critical to the nourishment and stability of the ocular structures.

The Pars Plana

The pars plana attaches to the ora serrata, the most anterior extension of the retina. It is continuous with the choroid posteriorly. The pars plana represents the anatomical landmark for accessing the posterior segment of the globe in vitreoretinal surgery.

Evaluation of the Ciliary Body

Because the ciliary processes produce aqueous, *tonometry* (a measurement of the intraocular pressure [IOP]) could be said to be an evaluation of their production capabilities. In truth, however, IOP is generally more a function of aqueous drainage (via the trabeculum, etc) rather than its production.

The ciliary muscle's involvement in accommodation cannot be measured directly. However, testing the patient's *amplitude of accommodation* gives a dioptric measurement of the patient's ability to change the focus of the crystalline lens in response to a near stimulus. The rigidity of the lens is considered to be more of a factor in accommodative amplitude than the function of the ciliary muscle.

The Aqueous

The aqueous (or, more classically, the "aqueous humor") is the watery fluid that occupies the AC and PC of the eye. It is produced by the ciliary processes at a rate of 2 to 2.5 microliters every minute. Its composition is similar, although not identical, to that of blood plasma (the liquid component of blood, minus all the blood cells).

The aqueous also contains the enzymes needed in the active secretion of the aqueous itself. Lactate is also present in the aqueous due to the metabolic activity of the cornea, lens, and other structures. In addition to contributing to corneal and lenticular metabolism, the aqueous is part of the optical pathway that light must take on its way to the retina. In its normal state, the aqueous is clear.

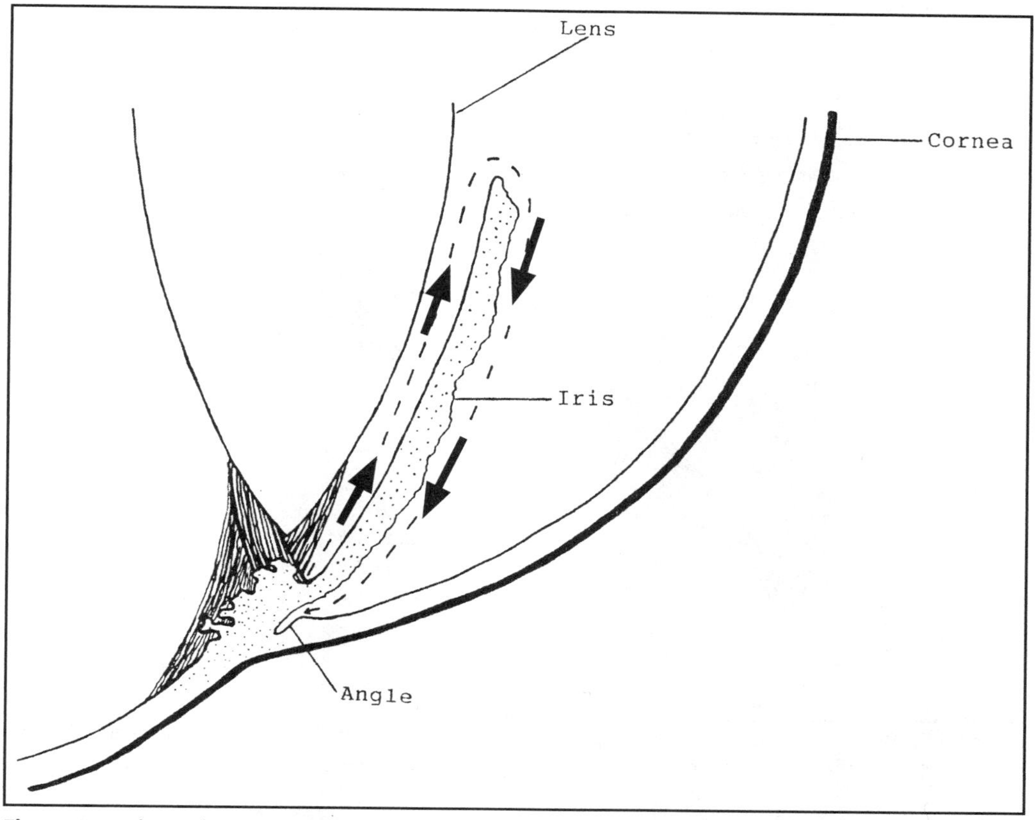

Figure 8-6. Flow of aqueous humor through the AC and PC. (Drawing by Holly Smith. Reprinted with permission from Gayton JL, Ledford JK. *The Crystal Clear Guide to Sight for Life*. Lancaster, PA: Starburst Publishers; 1996.)

Aqueous is formed in the PC and then circulates through the pupil into the AC (Figure 8-6). Hydrostatic and osmotic gradients assist in creating the circulation of the aqueous. The aqueous then leaves the eye through the angle (see next section).

The presence of the aqueous in the eye helps create a certain amount of resistance to sustain a constant shape of the ocular coat. It also creates the pressure within the eye. (This is also discussed in detail in a later section.) Some glaucoma medications lower IOP by decreasing the production of aqueous.

Evaluation of the Aqueous

The aqueous can be observed with the *slit lamp (biomicroscope)*. The normal aqueous is optically clear. If excessive protein (clinically termed *flare*) or blood cells (clinically termed *cell*) is present, it can generally be seen by pinpoint illumination. Larger amounts of blood and hyphema may be seen by direct illumination.

If it becomes necessary to evaluate the aqueous directly, an *AC tap* (or paracentesis) may be performed, in which a small amount of aqueous is removed from the eye using a needle and syringe. The fluid can then be analyzed for various components and entities, including antibodies, infectious agents, and different cell types.

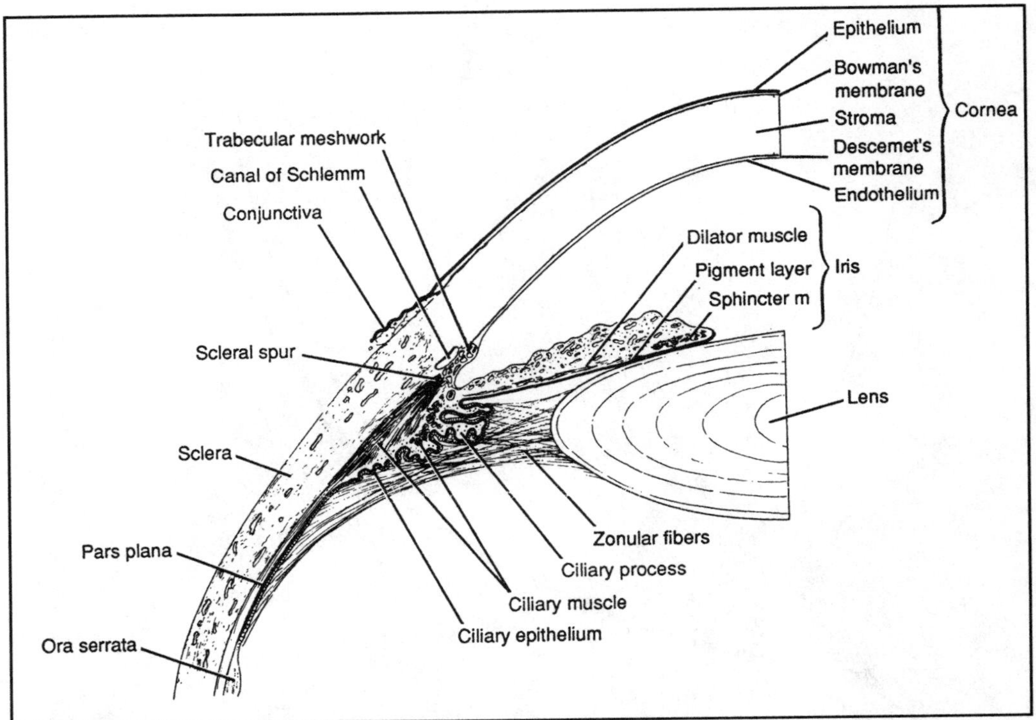

Figure 8-7. AC and related structures. (Reprinted with permission from Vaughan DG, Asbury T, Riordan-Eva P. *General Ophthalmology.* 13th ed. Norwalk, CT: Appleton and Lange; 1992.)

The Angle

The angle is the actual anatomical angle created by the root of the iris and the peripheral corneal vault (Figure 8-7). Within it lie the important structures involved in the outflow passages of aqueous, specifically the trabecular meshwork (TM) and canal of Schlemm (Figure 8-8).

The aqueous leaves the AC through the TM, a meshwork-like band lying just posterior to the peripheral corneal endothelium. Then the aqueous is collected in the canal of Schlemm, which is similar to a circular drain pipe with a small hole in its inner radius. The canal of Schlemm communicates peripherally with the angle's episcleral veins, which serve as the final drainage sites for the aqueous.

The relationship of the iris plane to the cornea (or angle opening) has a significant effect on the aqueous humor's accessibility to its outflow channels. If the iris and corneal endothelium have too small a separation or are "closed" against one another, the aqueous will not have access to the TM or canal of Schlemm for drainage (Figure 8-9). This is termed a *narrow angle*, and an eye with this configuration is at risk for an angle closure attack. (This will be discussed more fully under Evaluation of the Angle Structures on p. 76). The hyperopic (farsighted) eye is generally anatomically smaller, which means that the anterior segment is smaller and the angle opening narrower and thus more at risk for closure.

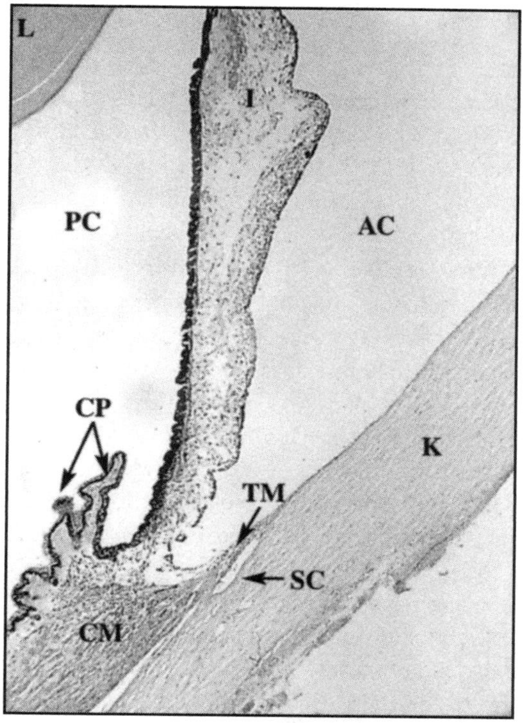

Figure 8-8. Microscopic section of an angle. L: lens; PC: posterior chamber; I: iris; CP: ciliary processes; CM: ciliary muscle; TM: trabecular meshwork; SC: Schlemm's canal; AC: anterior chamber; K: cornea. (Photo by Mark Greenwald, University of Tennessee—Memphis.)

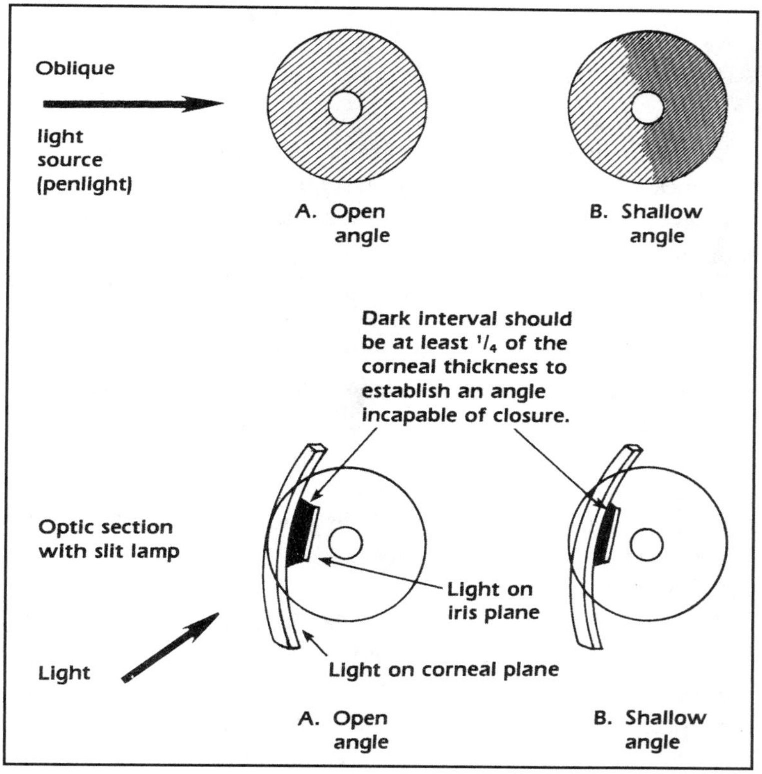

Figure 8-9. Techniques for assessing the angle opening. Top: penlight method. Bottom: slit lamp method. (Reprinted with permission from Nemeth SC, Shea CA. *Medical Sciences for the Ophthalmic Assistant.* Thorofare, NJ: SLACK Incorporated; 1988.)

Intraocular Pressure

IOP is created by the dynamics of the production of aqueous at the ciliary processes (inflow) and the drainage of aqueous through the TM to the canal of Schlemm (outflow). There is a normal physiologic balance between these dynamic forces. However, when these dynamics are disturbed and the inflow exceeds the outflow, the result is increased IOP.

IOP is measured with a *tonometer*. There are various types of tonometers, including applanation, indentation, noncontact, and the TonoPen (Intermedics Intraocular, Pasadena, CA) gives the pressure of the eye in millimeters of mercury (mm Hg). Normal IOP ranges from 10 to 21 mm Hg in the adult. If the IOP is too high, the pressure builds up and its forces are transferred toward the back of the eye. This leads to damage of the optic nerve with corresponding loss in the visual field. The triad of elevated IOP, nerve damage, and field loss are indicative of the disease glaucoma.

Patients whose pressures consistently stay over 21 mm Hg are termed *glaucoma suspects* or *ocular hypertensives*. However, the general population tolerates levels of pressure differently. While some people appear to develop damage with a normal IOP (normal or low tension glaucoma), others may not develop damage despite a significantly elevated IOP (suspects and hypertensives).

Contraction of the ciliary muscle also has effects on IOP. Pilocarpine, an older drug still sometimes used in the treatment of glaucoma, is thought to lower IOP through opening the pores in the TM by constricting and creating tension on the ciliary muscle.

For a full discussion on glaucoma, please refer to the Basic Bookshelf title *Cataracts and Glaucoma.*

Evaluation of the Angle Structures

An assessment of the angle and its structures is made with the *slit lamp* and a *gonioscopy lens*. The lens utilizes mirrors of different degrees of tilt, allowing one to view and analyze the relationships of the iris to the cornea, as well as the TM and canal of Schlemm (Figure 8-10). The angle is assessed on a common grading system. A grade 4 signifies the greatest degree of angle ("wide open"), while a grade 1 represents the smallest degree of angle ("narrow angle"). Grades are based on which structures are visible with the gonioscope, as the TM will not be visible with narrower angles.

Angle estimation techniques are also used to evaluate the openness or narrowness of the angle. A *penlight* may be used to grossly estimate the iris/cornea relationship. Viewing an "open" angle with a "deep" chamber, a penlight held at the limbal area will illuminate the entire iris, causing light to be dispersed evenly. Viewing a "narrow" angle with a "shallow" chamber, the light held from the temporal side will cast a shadow on the nasal side due to iris convexity. It is similar to comparing the sun shining on a flat, open field where light is dispersed (deep chamber) or the sun shining on a mountain where light is caught on one side and in the shadows on the opposite side (narrow chamber) (see Figure 8-9, top).

The *slit lamp* can also be used to assess this relationship. The "dark interval" between the corneal reflex light and iris plane light represents the depth of the AC (see Figure 8-9, bottom). For the angle to be considered open, this dark interval should be approximately one-quarter of the corneal width at the corneal periphery. If it is less than this, one is viewing a narrow angle.

Estimation of angles is of vital importance if the patient is to be dilated. Dilating a patient with a narrow angle may cause the iris to bunch up against the lens, blocking off the flow of

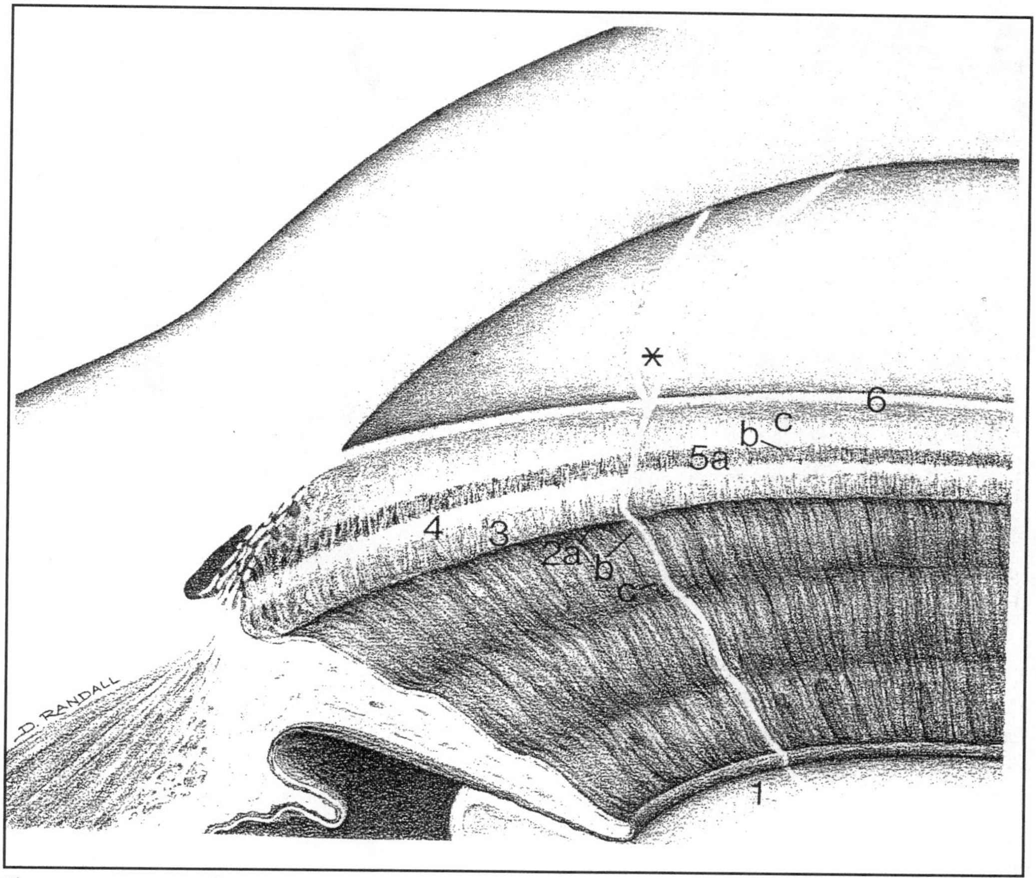

Figure 8-10. AC angle as seen through a gonio lens. (1) Pupillary border; (2) Peripheral iris a-insertion, b-curvature, c-angular approach; (3) Ciliary body band; (4) Scleral spur; (5) TM, a-posterior, b-mid, c-anterior; (6) Schwalbe's line; (*) Corneal optical wedge. (Reprinted with permission from Fellman Rl, Spaeth GL, Starita RJ. Gonioscopy: key to successful management of glaucoma. *Clinical Modules for Ophthalmologists*. San Francisco, CA: American Academy of Ophthalmology; 1984.)

aqueous humor. Because the aqueous cannot drain, pressure rapidly builds up inside the eye. This scenario is known as an angle closure attack. The high pressure causes pain, redness, and corneal edema (resulting in blurred vision and/or halos around lights). If sustained long enough, the pressure can cause irreversible damage to the optic nerve. Thus, angle closure is a true ocular emergency.

IOP fluctuates during a 24-hour period (diurnal variation), with peak pressure occurring about midday. Many times the physician will want to check the patient's pressure at different times of the day and will thus schedule a patient for an IOP check at a specific time. Sometimes a study will be done to document a patient's IOPs through the night for nocturnal data.

The Lens

The lens is the transparent biconvex intraocular structure that actively participates in the functions of accommodation and refraction. In medical terminology, the combining form phaco- (or

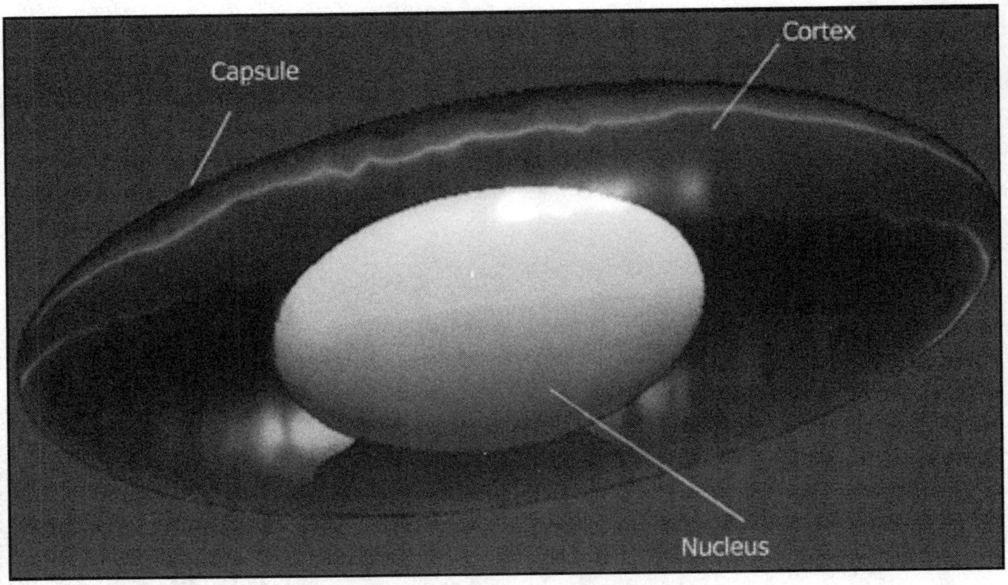

Figure 8-11. Layers of the lens. (Illustration by Stephanie Embrey.)

phako-) denotes the lens. Thus a phakic eye is one having the natural lens; aphakic means that the lens has been removed, and pseudophakia denotes the presence of an artificial lens (as in an intraocular lens (IOL) implant inserted following surgical removal of the lens, discussed later).

The lens is located directly behind the iris. Fine zonular fibers originating from the ciliary body (pars plicata portion) attach to the lens, suspending it behind the pupil. Anteriorly, it is bathed in aqueous; posteriorly, it lies against the vitreous. The lens possesses no innervation or blood supply after fetal development. Anatomically it has three distinct parts: the capsule, the epithelium, and the lens substance (the cortex and nucleus) (Figure 8-11).

The capsule is an elastic membrane that envelops the entire lens. During cataract surgery (discussed in a moment), the anterior capsule is opened and the inner cortex and nucleus removed. The posterior two-thirds of the capsule are left intact to support an artificial lens implant. Sometimes the remaining capsule becomes cloudy (misnamed secondary or after cataract, and more properly called posterior capsule opacity) and the patient's vision once again decreases. This situation is easily remedied by creating an opening in the center of the capsule membrane with a laser, clearing the pathway for light and improving sight.

The epithelium is located directly under the lens capsule. A single layer of cells grow and migrate toward the equator of the lens. The cells elongate, creating new lens fibers that constantly add to the lens substance throughout life.

The lens can be divided into stratified zones, which represent the order (timeline) the lens fibers were laid down. Remember how a tree grows? The inner rings represent the first growth of the tree. The lens is constructed similarly. Under the slit lamp these zones have different light appearances due to their different indices of refractions.

The nucleus (center) of the lens actually contains many different nuclei, differentiated by time of development. Beginning in the center and moving outward, there is the embryonic, fetal, infantile, and adult nuclei. At the level of the fetal nucleus are several fine lines (sutures) in the shape of a Y. Those sutures represent fiber growth at that stage in development. The anterior Y is upright, while the posterior Y is inverted.

The cortex is made of young soft fibers that lie beneath the lens capsule. It possesses the highest concentration of water within the lens.

The metabolism of the lens and the removal of its waste products are performed by the surrounding aqueous and vitreous. The lens is rather unique in that it continues to grow throughout life without shedding any of its cellular material. Cells are constantly being produced internally; consequently, the lens becomes more compact over time.

A cataract represents an opacity of the lens tissue that can result from any metabolic insult to the lens. The lens undergoes metabolic changes with aging, thus normal age-related degeneration is the most common cause of cataracts. Less frequently, cataracts may be caused by chemical (usually from medications), electrical, or radiation toxicity, as well as mechanical damage (trauma). When the opacity evolves to the point of interfering with vision, the cataract is surgically removed. Currently, the most common technique for removal of the cortex and nucleus is phacoemulsification (or "phaco" for short). After the capsule is opened as described earlier, the lens material is emulsified with ultrasound and then suctioned out through a small tubule. The posterior capsule surface is polished and an artificial lens (IOL implant, or IOL) is placed in front of the capsule.

Cataracts are categorized by several criteria. Congenital, juvenile, and senile describe cataracts by the age at which they appear. Alternately, lens opacities might be listed according to their cause (diabetic, glass-blower's, traumatic, etc). The appearance of the cataract may also be used to classify (brunescent, black, etc). A cataract may also be designated by its stage (early, incipient, mature, etc).

Probably the most common designation is by the part of the lens affected (cortical, nuclear, subcapsular, etc.). Nuclear sclerosis (NS) and posterior subcapsular cataracts (PSCs) are among the most common types of cataracts seen clinically.

The lens possesses about +16 diopters of the total dioptric power of the eye. The lens obeys the laws of optics: light is bent or refracted at the interface between two areas of different indices of refraction. It has an index of refraction of 1.42, which is greater than the surrounding aqueous and vitreous. During the aging process and following metabolic insults, the index of refraction of the lens changes.

When the eye is in a relaxed state, both the lens shape and index of refraction converge parallel rays from a distant object onto the retina. When viewing a near object, the lens must shorten its focal length in order to keep the image clear on the retina (accommodation).

The total amount of dioptric change the lens produces by changing its shape is called the amplitude of accommodation. This ability to change shape in the lens is greatest during childhood when the lens is more pliable. The amplitude decreases with age as the lens loses its flexibility, leveling off at about 55 years old. A child can hold an object very close and focus on it, while a person in his or her 40s has to hold the object at arm's length for clear viewing. This occurs because the lens has lost "plus" power and its focal point has shifted back. (Accommodation is discussed in Chapter 15.)

Evaluation of the Lens

The *slit lamp* is ideal for evaluating the layers of the lens: anterior capsule, cortex, nucleus, and posterior capsule. This is best done through a dilated pupil. Direct illumination (shining the light right onto the lens, Figure 8-12A) or retroillumination (using light reflected off the retina to back-illuminate the lens, Figure 8-12B) may be used.

With the *direct ophthalmoscope*, using a spot beam at +8.00-diopter to +10.0-diopter setting, the optical clarity of the media, including the lens, can be checked. A cataract might also

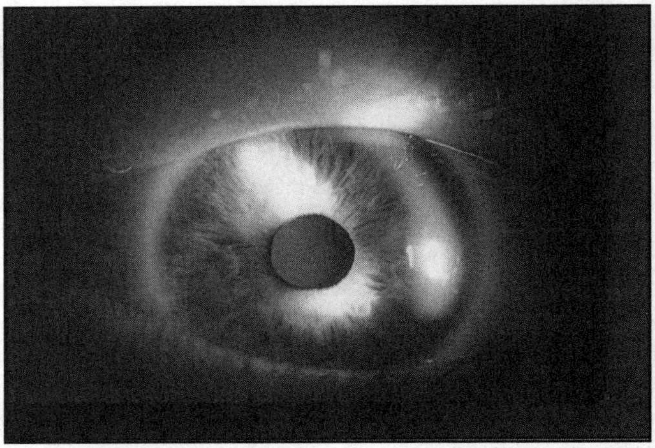

Figure 8-12A. Slit lamp view of the lens. (Photo by Val Sanders. Reprinted with permission from Ledford JK, Sanders VN. *The Slit Lamp Primer, Second Edition*. Thorofare, NJ: SLACK Incorporated; 2006.)

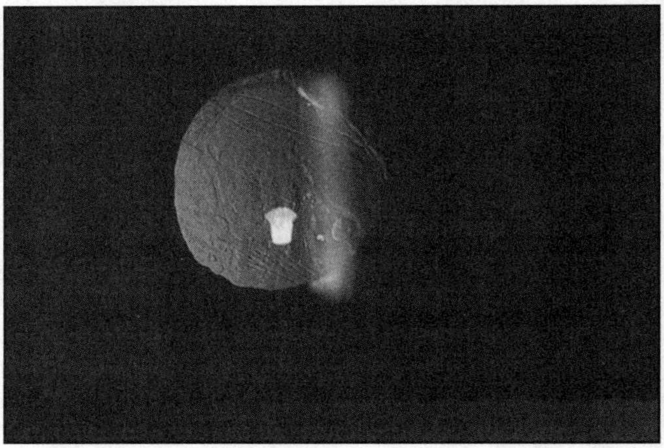

Figure 8-12B. Retroillumination of the lens. (Photo by Val Sanders. Reprinted with permission from Ledford JK, Sanders VN. *The Slit Lamp Primer, Second Edition*. Thorofare, NJ: SLACK Incorporated; 2006.)

be seen with the retinoscope, although this is not an instrument designed to specifically evaluate the lens.

While contrast sensitivity testing (CST) is actually a retinal test, it is often used as an indicator of the visual interference caused by a lens opacity. Standard Snellen acuity charts are high contrast, and a patient may read 20/20 yet be visually impaired. In real life, this can translate to debilitating loss of vision in low-contrast situations (fog, for example). On the other hand, brightness may also be an issue in cataracts. In this case, light coming into the eye is scattered or the pupil is constricted so that the patient is looking through the densest part of the cataract. Glare testing can show the difference between Snellen acuity and the vision under bright light conditions (simulating direct sun and car lights at night).

Glossary of Common Disorders

angle closure glaucoma: Acute glaucoma attack in which aqueous humor is physically blocked internally from draining out of the AC, causing a sudden rise of pressure in the eye; hallmarks are redness, pain, and blurred vision (including halos around lights).

anisocoria: Situation in which the pupils are not of equal size.

anterior uveitis/iritis: Inflammation of the iris and/or ciliary body.

Argyll Robertson pupil*: Condition in which a pupil constricts upon accommodation but does not react to varying direct or consensual light; usually associated with syphilis.

cataract: Any opacity in the crystalline lens; there are many types, classified by age of onset, appearance, cause, location in the lens, etc.

exfoliation syndrome*: Condition in which flakes of ocular and somatic material appear on structures in the AC, including the TM, where they may block aqueous outflow and cause a rise in IOP (pseudoexfoliative glaucoma); while "true" exfoliation in the eye is considered to occur within the crystalline lens itself, in ophthalmic usage, this term usually describes exfoliation/pseudoexfoliation syndrome in which flakes appear on the lens; also called pseudoexfoliation syndrome.

glaucoma: A group of disorders characterized by IOP that damages the optic nerve.

heterochromia iridis: Condition in which the irises are different colors, or there is more than one color in a single iris.

Horner's syndrome*: Disorder of the third cranial nerve causing miosis, ptosis, and anhidrosis (lack of sweating) on the affected side.

hyphema: Presence of blood in the AC.

hypopyon: Presence of purulent material (ie, white blood cells or pus) in the AC.

iris coloboma*: Partial absence of or gap in the iris, usually in the lower half of the structure and usually a result of incomplete fusion of fetal tissue

Marcus Gunn pupil (also called afferent pupillary defect and relative afferent pupillary defect)*: Impairment of the normal response of the affected pupil to bright light; usually appears as a constriction of both pupils when the unaffected eye is illuminated, followed by an apparent dilation of both pupils when the affected eye is illuminated.

narrow angles: Anatomical situation in which the angle between the iris and cornea of the eye is abnormally narrow, increasing the likelihood of an angle-closure glaucoma attack.

pseudoexfoliation syndrome: Another term for exfoliation syndrome.

synechia: Adhesions of the iris to either the posterior corneal surface (anterior synechia) or the anterior lens surface (posterior synechia); usually seen in inflammatory disorders.

tonic pupil (also called Adie's pupil or Adie's syndrome, myotonic or tonic pupil)*: Uneven contraction of the pupils of each eye upon accommodation (in near vision) in which the affected pupil reacts poorly to light and slowly to near.

* These definitions are used with permission from Ledford JK, Hoffman J. *Quick Reference Dictionary of Eyecare Terminology, Fifth Edition.* Thorofare, NJ: SLACK Incorporated; 2008.

Chapter 9

The Posterior Segment

Sheila Coyne Nemeth, COMT

Carolyn Shea, COMT

Mark DiSclafani, MD

Mark Schluter, MD

KEY POINTS

- The posterior segment includes the vitreous, posterior sclera, choroid, retina, and optic nerve.
- The choroid is a dense network of blood vessels sandwiched between the retina and sclera. It provides nourishment to the photoreceptors (rods and cones) and the retinal pigment epithelium (RPE). The choroid is the posterior part of the uvea (other uveal tissue is the iris and ciliary body).
- The retina contains the photochemicals (ie, rhodopsin) and the neurologic connections (rods, cones, and ganglion cells) that process light energy and relay it via the optic nerve to our visual cortex for visual perception and integration.
- The macula is 1.5 mm of the central retina. It surrounds the fovea, which is approximately 500 μm in diameter and the site from which our most detailed vision originates.
- The photoreceptor cells of the retina are the rods and cones. The rods, numbering 130 million, are responsible for peripheral and scotopic (low luminance) vision. The cones, numbering 6 million, provide both color vision and the ability to see detail and fine resolution.

The Vitreous

The vitreous fills the large cavity behind the lens of the eye (Figure 9-1). It is actually about 99% water. The vitreous has a small amount of collagen in it, giving it the consistency of a gel. It is clear and avascular and contributes approximately two-thirds of the volume and weight of the eye. It functions as an optically transparent medium to transmit light bent by the cornea and lens. The vitreous also gives volume and form to the globe; lack of vitreous can cause the globe to shrink and collapse. Unlike aqueous humor, the vitreous is not continually reformed or resupplied. When the eye reaches adult size, vitreous formation is complete and the adult lives with this amount of vitreous throughout life.

The formed vitreous shrinks with age, like a gel pulling away from the edges of a bowl. The body secretes fluid into the newly vacant space, making the vitreous more fluid-like and less gel-like (a degenerative process known as syneresis). During this process the vitreous may become detached from the back of the eye (vitreous detachment). When this occurs, the patient may complain of seeing many floaters, flashes of light, or both.

Floaters are small opacities (clumps of pigment or protein) in the vitreous. Since the vitreous is one of the clear refracting mediums of the ocular system, any "solid" or "opaque" object within the vitreous (such as a pigmented floater) casts a shadow onto the retina. This creates the visual symptom of "specks." They can be noticed most easily when the patient looks at a uniform light-colored background, such as the blue sky. They do not affect the visual acuity, and sometimes settle down in the inferior peripheral vitreous where they are no longer perceived.

Floaters are most often signs of the natural aging of the globe, yet younger myopes may have this condition also. However, a sudden new onset of floaters with a "curtain" coming down in one part of the field of vision is a serious complaint, as these can be symptoms of a retinal detachment (RD). This detachment can occur due to the traction of the vitreous pulling on the retina, causing a hole in the retina and subsequent detachment. Floaters, therefore, constitute an important symptom indicating the need for a full ophthalmologic examination. Light flashes, which usually appear in the temporal field of vision, are commonly described as "lightning streaks." They are also caused by the vitreous gel pulling on the retina. Because of the close relationship of the vitreous and retina, many retinal disorders are now termed *vitreoretinal diseases*.

The vitreous is subject to infection and inflammation from exogenous (outside the body) or endogenous organisms (inside the body). The vitreous is an excellent culture medium for anaerobic (not requiring air) bacteria or fungi, and infection can cause a diffuse and severe reaction termed *bacterial endophthalmitis*. The vitreous may also be affected by internal bleeding (vitreous hemorrhage), cholesterol crystal aggregates (syneresis scintillans), and calcium soap deposits (asteroid hyalosis). Because the vitreous is part of the optical media, anything that reduces its transparency (such as blood) causes a decrease in vision.

Evaluation of the Vitreous

The anterior vitreous can be examined through a dilated pupil by utilizing a slit beam from the *biomicroscope* (slit lamp) and sectioning through the vitreous. A variety of abnormalities can be noted in this way. The presence of blood, pigment, or inflammatory cells allow the organization of the normally fine fibrillar strands to be appreciated. The gel may become diffusely stained by long-standing hemorrhage. The vitreous is typically somewhat mobile when the eye moves. The slit lamp can also be used to observe any increase or decrease in this mobility.

The *78 or 90 diopter lens* is a small, powerful convex lens that is hand-held in front of the patient's dilated pupil while the examiner looks through the biomicroscope. This lens affords a

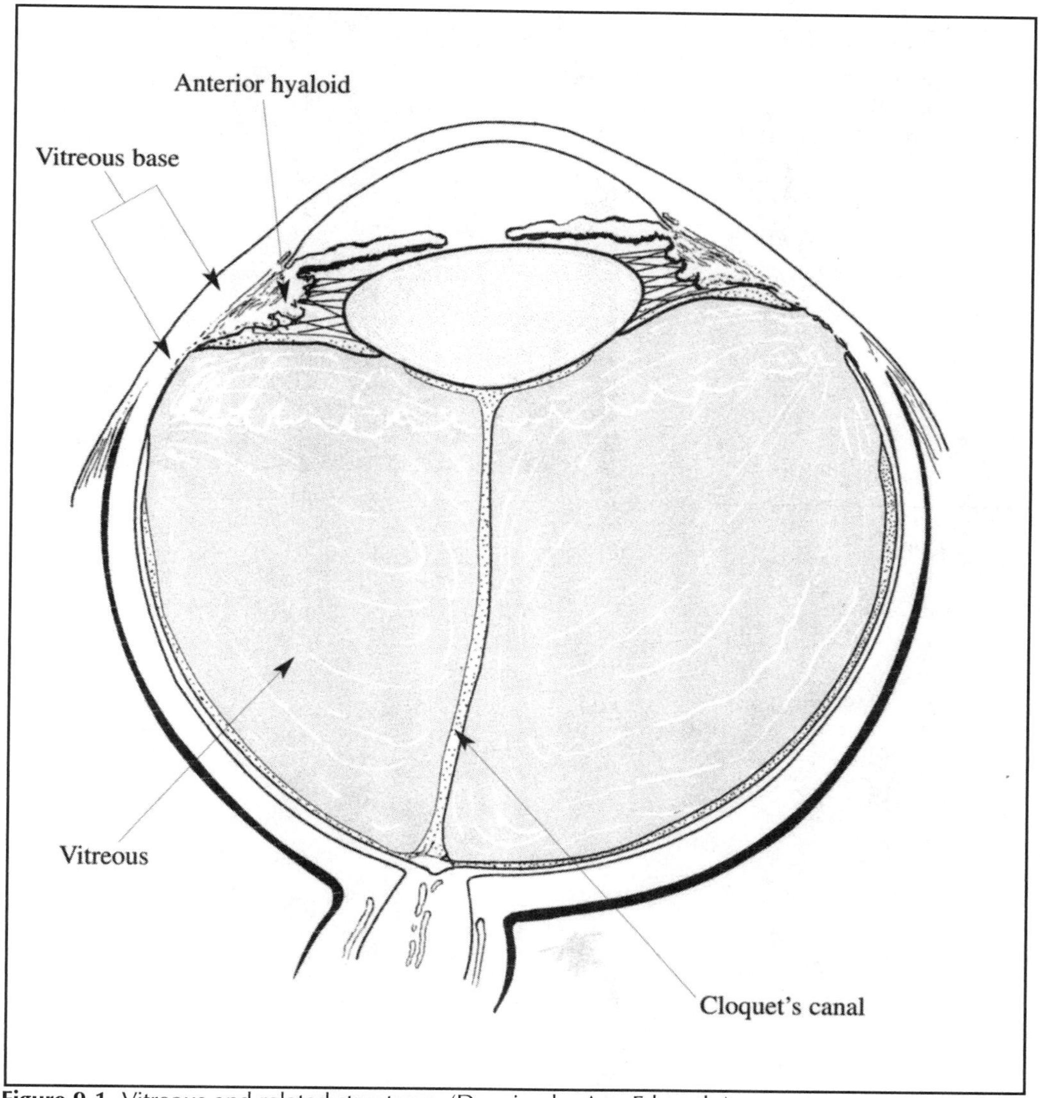

Figure 9-1. Vitreous and related structures. (Drawing by Ana Edwards.)

stereoscopic view of the posterior segment, including the posterior vitreous, retina, and optic disk. It is very useful in the examination of the vitreoretinal interface and in the detection of macular disease or pathologic cupping (glaucoma).

Indirect ophthalmoscopy also allows the examiner a stereoscopic wide-angle view of essentially the entire retina, including the far periphery. By performing *scleral depression* during the examination, fine details of the peripheral vitreoretinal interface such as adhesions, thinning, or small retinal breaks can be seen.

B-scan ultrasonography is an excellent tool in evaluating the vitreous. The normal vitreous is an acoustics-free space, and sound penetrates it without reflective interference (echoes). Abnormal echoes of varying amplitudes can be seen in vitreous hemorrhages, asteroid hyalosis (Figure 9-2), syneresis scintillans, or vitreous inflammation (vitritis). B-scan is frequently used to rule out a RD when a severe vitreous hemorrhage does not allow direct visualization of the retina.

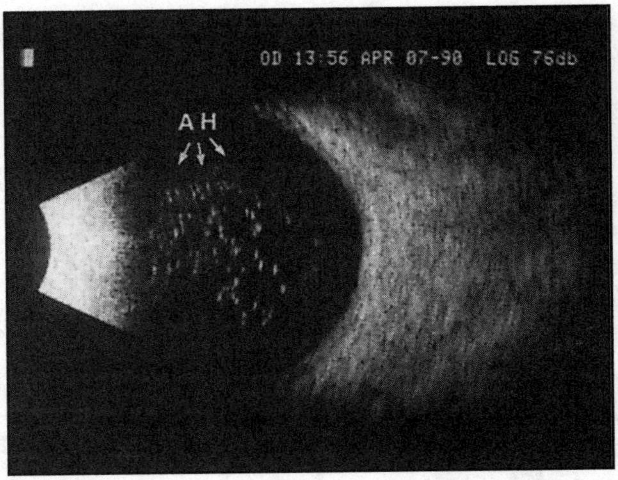

Figure 9-2. B-scan showing asteroid hyalosis (AH) in the vitreous. (Reprinted with permission from Kendall CJ. *Ophthalmic Echography*. Thorofare, NJ: SLACK Incorporated; 1990.)

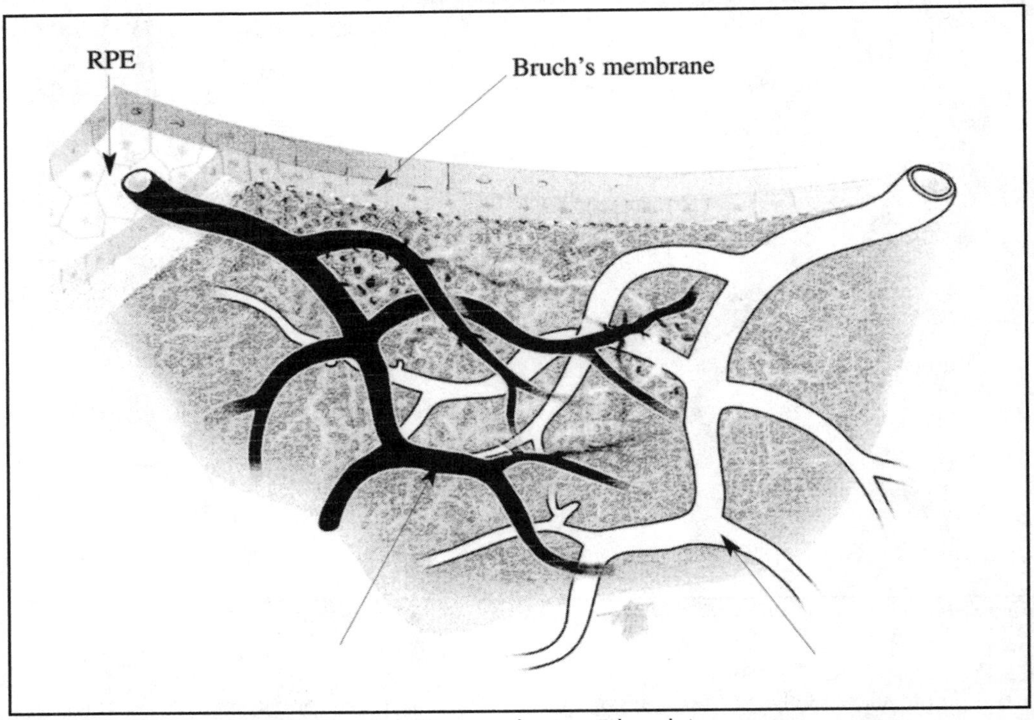

Figure 9-3. Vasculature of the choroid. (Drawing by Ana Edwards.)

Choroid

The choroid is a large network of blood vessels lying between the retina and sclera (Figure 9-3). The choroid nourishes the outer layers of the retina, including the all-important photoreceptors (rods and cones) and the RPE.

The choroid is part of the uvea, along with the iris and ciliary body. As uvea means "grape" in Latin, the name is indicative of the deep blue tones that this vascular tract can give to the sclera, as with episodes of scleral inflammation (scleritis).

The choroid is attached to the margin of the optic nerve and extends to the ora serrata and then joins with the ciliary body. The choroid receives its arterial blood supply from three different branches of the ophthalmic artery: the long and short posterior ciliary arteries and the anterior ciliary arteries. The short posterior ciliary arteries supply the most posterior portion of the choroid. Although both the retina and the choroid receive their blood supply from one source (the ophthalmic artery), these two blood supplies are quite separate in function. The choroidal blood vessels can be divided into two categories: 1) the fine capillaries that represent the innermost layer of the choroidal vessels (the choriocapillaris), and 2) the larger caliber arteries and veins that lie just posterior to the choriocapillaris (these can easily be seen in an albino fundus because there is minimal pigment obscuring the vessels).

The veins in each quadrant of the choroid connect together to form a vortex vein. There is thus one vortex vein in each quadrant of the posterior retina. The vortex veins represent surgical landmarks and also nightmares—as piercing one of them causes profuse bleeding. They are also sensitive areas when applying laser treatment, as patients tend to feel the laser more when it is applied near these areas because there is a nerve supply close by.

Bruch's membrane is a semipermeable membrane that lies on top of (anterior to) the choriocapillaris and at the bottom of the RPE layer of the retina. It is known as a "basement membrane." This membrane allows nutrients to pass from the choriocapillaris to the outer layers of the retina and serves as a sieve when retinal debris attempts to leave through the pores in the choriocapillaris vessels. Retinal drusen (small, round, yellowing lesions commonly seen in older individuals) are thought to be by-products excreted by the RPE just above Bruch's membrane (ie, a buildup of "trash" that did not make it to the choriocapillaris). Angioid streaks represent splits, or "cracks," in Bruch's membrane and appear as reddish-brown streaks radiating from the optic disk. They are associated with diseases that affect the elastic tissue of the body.

There are many systemic diseases that cause insult to the choroid and the retina, resulting in chorioretinitis. Diseases associated with chorioretinitis include toxoplasmosis, syphilis, histoplasmosis, tuberculosis, and sarcoidosis. *Uveitis* is the term used to describe inflammation of the uveal tract, but it does not specify where in the tract the condition is occurring. Anterior uveitis is most commonly referred to as iritis, while posterior uveitis is most commonly called choroiditis or (when involving both choroid and retina) chorioretinitis.

Evaluation of the Choroid

The "prearterial phase" of *fluorescein angiography* is the filling of the choroidal vessels. The filling of these vessels is rather segmented and patchy due to the choriocapillaris' rather lobular network design. Dye reaches the choroidal network before the central retinal artery, thus the network appears on the "earlies" of the run. The dye from the choriocapillaris stains the sclera, which is seen as a mottled background fluorescence during the sequenced angiographic run.

Recent advances in digital imaging with *indocyanine-green* (ICG) cameras have allowed clinicians to directly visualize the choroidal vasculature for the first time. Intravenous sodium fluorescein dye, the most commonly used dye for diagnostic retinal studies, has poor transmission of fluorescence through fundus pigmentation. ICG dye absorbs and emits light in the near-infrared range. This dye maximally fluoresces at 835 nm; these long wavelengths penetrate through ocular pigment (ie, the RPE) much more efficiently than the shorter wavelengths of fluorescein dye. Localization and detection of the abnormal choroidal vessels that occur in "wet" age-related maculopathy (ARM) makes ICG dye a useful clinical tool.

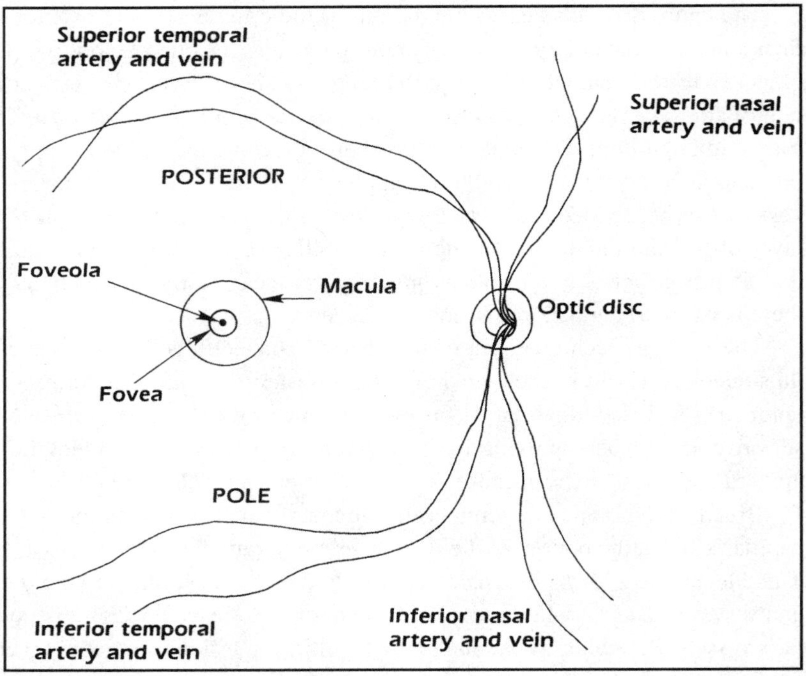

Figure 9-4. Schematic of macula and its relationship to the posterior pole. (Reprinted with permission from Nemeth SC, Shea CA. *Medical Sciences for the Ophthalmic Assistant.* Thorofare, NJ: SLACK Incorporated; 1988.)

The Retina

The transparent neural tissue lining the posterior two-thirds of the eye is the retina: the "color film" of our visual system. Without the retina, all visual sense is lost. The retina contains the photochemicals and neurologic connections that process light energy and relay it to our visual cortex for visual perception and integration.

Macula and Fovea

The macula is 1.5 mm of the central retina, surrounding the fovea (which is approximately 500 μm in diameter). The fovea of the retina represents the center, or peak, of clearest vision and the site of our most detailed color vision; it can be thought of as the top of the mountain. It has as its center, or the very tip of the mountain, the foveola. Clinically, the macula is sometimes referred to as the "posterior pole," or the area lying between the "arcades" (areas inside the main branches of the central retinal artery and vein) (Figure 9-4). When viewing the macula with a fundus camera or an ophthalmoscope, one can see a yellowish reflex in the macula area due to the presence of xanthophyll, a yellow pigment. The color of this reflex has led to the macula being referred to as the macula lutea (yellow macula). The normal macula appears darker than the rest of the retina because of the xanthophyll and because the RPE in the macular area contains more melanin. Also, the macula has no nerve fiber layer (NFL), which allows the light direct access to the rods and cones underneath. Finally, the distribution of different types of cone axons (X and Y cells) are predominantly in the center, allowing color perception and contrast sensitivity. (We will discuss the rods and cones more later.)

Senile macular degeneration (SMD), now called age-related macular degeneration (ARMD), is a relatively common cause of acquired central visual loss in the elderly. ARMD is caused by degeneration, or breakdown, in the RPE layer of the retina. Symptoms include words appearing blurry on a page of text, straight lines looking distorted, or a dark "cut out" hole in the center of vision. Color vision may also become dimmer. A less common type is exudative (or "wet") ARMD in which aberrant blood vessels grow into the macular area and leak. These vessels may also bleed under or into the retina, destroying central vision.

Other Landmarks

The vortex veins are veins in each quadrant of the midperipheral retina that serve to drain the retina. The ora serrata is the anterior termination of the retina. The ora is patterned in a serrated fashion and meets the pars plana of the ciliary body. The vitreous is very tightly fused to the peripheral retina near the ora serrata.

Retinal Layers

The retina is composed of two basic layers: the outer (more posterior) RPE layer and the inner neurosensory layer. There is a "potential space" between the inner neurosensory retina and the outer RPE. The cause of many retinal detachments (RDs) is a tear in the retina where fluid passes through the hole and between the photoreceptors (rods and cones) and the RPE. (These holes can be caused by the vitreous tugging at the retina or by inherent weaknesses in the retina.) The subretinal fluid is actually liquefied vitreous that passes through the hole and creates a pool of fluid beneath the inner layer, causing separation and detachment. This type of RD is termed a *rhegmatogenous detachment*. It can be surgically treated by first "sealing" the hole with heat or cryo (freezing), then a silicone scleral buckle is placed around the globe, acting as a mechanical "girdle" that folds the outer wall of the eye inward to touch the inner layers, thus reinstating the normal anatomical relationships for proper functioning.

Symptoms of RDs include a sudden onset of floaters, flashes of "streaking light," and shadows or curtains coming across the visual field. The visual acuity may or may not be decreased, depending on whether or not the macula has been detached.

The retina can be further divided into the nine layers of the sensory retina and the one layer of outer pigment layer (Figure 9-5). We will discuss the layers, starting from the scleral/choroidal/Bruch's membrane side and proceed to the "inner" layers that oppose the vitreous. As you study these layers, keep in mind that the entire retina is only 0.5 mm thick.

Retinal Pigment Epithelium

The RPE is a highly pigmented layer that absorbs excess light. When one looks at the color of the fundus, one is actually looking at the color and patterning of this layer, not the other nine layers (which are transparent). The color of this pigment is genetically determined. Blondes and redheads have minimal pigment in the RPE layer and thus the larger vessels of the choroid, lying posterior to the RPE, are readily evident. Brunettes have much heavier pigment and exhibit a so-called tigroid (brown and orange-pink) fundus, while albinos have no pigment at all. Asians and Indians have a bluish-black RPE. The variations of fundus color, vascular structure, and the optic disk are so exceedingly individualized that a security company has recently made a fundus scanning device for top security identification. Our fundus patterns are as unique as our fingerprints!

The RPE serves as a nourishing and garbage-collecting layer for the photoreceptors. It also functions as a "pump" for the sensory retina, exerting an adhesive force for the critical physiologic juxtaposition of the RPE and the photoreceptors. The RPE cells have very tight junctions between themselves, which prevents diffusion of substances between the choroidal

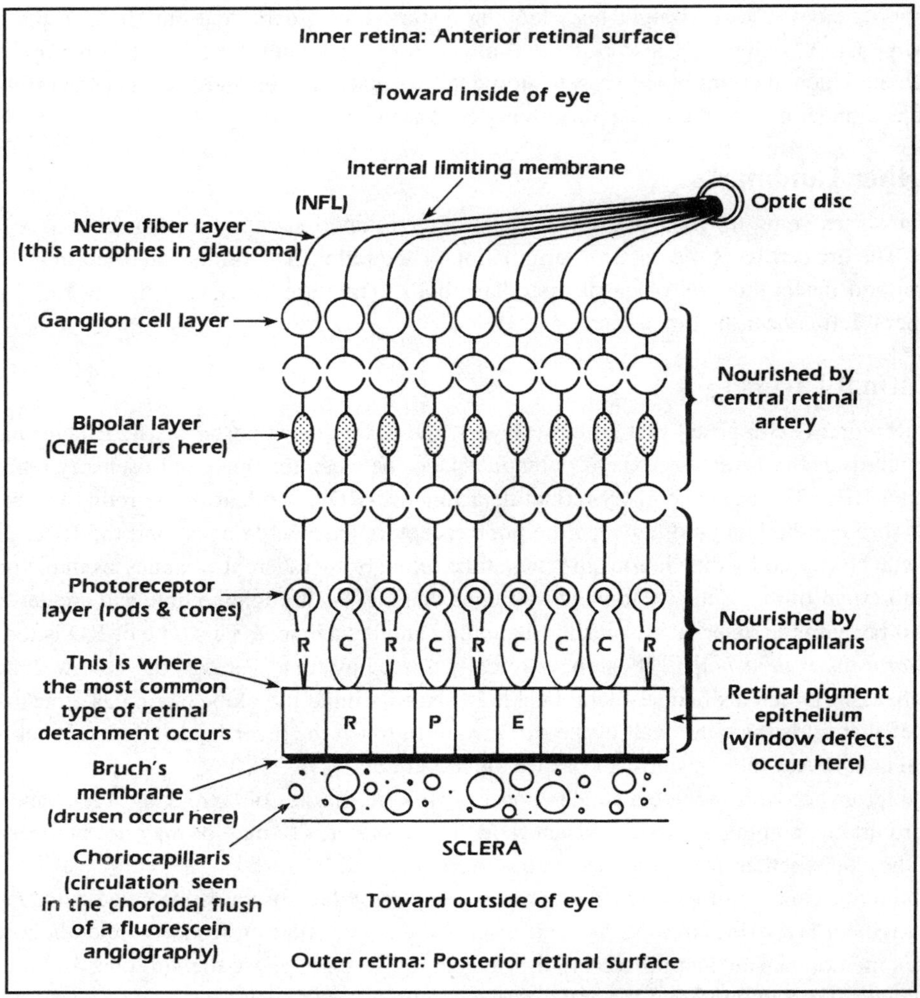

Figure 9-5. Schematic of retinal anatomy. (Reprinted with permission from Nemeth SC, Shea CA. *Medical Sciences for the Ophthalmic Assistant.* Thorofare, NJ: SLACK Incorporated; 1988.)

circulation and the retina. In fluorescein angiography of the retina, the prearterial phase (choroidal flush phase) tests the effectiveness of the RPE's tight junctions. If there is an absence (with disease) of the RPE, the RPE fails to block the fluorescein and an area of hyperfluorescence appears fairly early in the films. This is termed a *transmission defect* or a *window defect.*

The Three Vital Neural Transmitters

There are three important layers of the retina that serve as the key elements in the transmission of the nerve impulse to the brain: the photoreceptor layer (rods and cones), the bipolar layer, and the ganglion cell layer with its NFL.

The Photoreceptor Layer

The highly specialized cells known as the photoreceptors are responsible for converting light energy (electromagnetic energy) into nerve impulses. There are two specialized types of photoreceptors: the rods and cones, so named for their microscopic appearance. The approximate ratio of rods to cones is 20:1. The RPE, just posterior to the rods and cones, nourishes these critical cells. The rods and cones are capable of converting electromagnetic radiation energy of approximately 400 to 700 nm in wavelength into nerve impulses. These wavelengths represent the spectrum of "visible light." Ultraviolet light is outside of the spectrum of visual light. The retina is actually capable of seeing this wavelength, but the cornea and lens filter it out. After the lens has been removed, as in cataract surgery, some ultraviolet light can reach the retina. There has been much research into ultraviolet effects on the macula. Consequently, manufacturers of IOLs have developed polymers with ultraviolet-absorbing properties.

The Rods and Night Vision

There are approximately 130 million rods in the retina. They are primarily concerned with night vision or vision in dim illumination. This is termed *scotopic vision.* The majority of rods are in the periphery of the retina and are thus responsible for peripheral vision. After adaptation in the dark, the peripheral retina becomes most sensitive to light. The rods have been found to be most sensitive to blue (500 nm) light. At dusk, as the eye is adapting to the dark, the rods are being switched "on" and more messages are being sent to the blue hue center in the brain. Therefore, blues and greens will appear brighter than reds and yellows at nightfall. This is termed the *Purkinje effect.*

The key to the rods' ability to convert light to impulses is the visual pigment known as rhodopsin, contained within the rod receptor. Through a complex chain of chemical changes activated by light, rhodopsin begins the events that produce the nerve impulse. Rhodopsin is capable of absorbing specific wavelengths of visible light, which activates the very beginning of the photochemical reaction of the visual pathway. Rhodopsin is regenerated in the dark. Total dark adaptation, which would be a complete regeneration of rhodopsin, takes approximately 30 minutes. Clinical measurement of dark adaptation is a useful tool in the diagnosis of congenital rod malfunctioning, known as congenital stationary night blindness (CSNB).

Vitamin A is an essential component of rhodopsin. Deficiency of vitamin A can lead to night blindness due to the insufficient amount of rhodopsin produced. This deficiency primarily occurs in underdeveloped countries with dietary imbalances. It is reversible when treated.

Retinitis pigmentosa is an inherited retinal dystrophy that mainly affects the rod cells. A defect in rod metabolism causes night blindness and eventually a closing in of the peripheral visual field.

The Cones and Color Vision

There are approximately 6 million cones in the retina. Cones are clustered predominantly in the macula, and they provide both color vision and central, fine vision. Cones function best in photopic conditions (full illumination). Due to the high number of cones in the macula (and the relative absence of rods), color vision testing is basically a test of macular and optic nerve function.

The retina has at least three different kinds of cones, each kind having a different visual pigment that absorbs a specific wavelength of light. The three kinds of cones are red, green, and blue. The red cones contain the pigment erythrolabe, which absorbs light best at wavelength 570 nm. The green cones contain the pigment chlorolabe and have maximum sensitivity at 540 nm. The blue cones contain cyanolabe, absorbing 440 nm the best. All other colors we perceive are a result of the relative stimulation of the three pigments. Normal color vision occurs in 92% of the population. People with normal color vision are known as trichromats. Along with normal concentrations of these three cone pigments, trichromats must have normal "wiring" in the retina for visual processing.

The most common type of color deficit is the anomalous trichromat: the person who has all three cone pigments, but one pigment functions below standard. If the red is deficient, the person is protanomalous; if green is deficient, the person is deuteranomalous; and if the blue is deficient, the person is tritanomalous. Anomalous trichromats see a desaturated spectrum ("washed out") and have poor hue discrimination (need greater than normal changes in wavelength to tell a hue change). All three pigments are present, but one is deficient. Most anomalous trichromats confuse red and green, therefore termed *red/green color blindness*. This occurs in approximately 8% of Caucasian males and 0.5% of females, because it has a sex-linked recessive pattern of inheritance. The females are the genetic carriers, while the males manifest the characteristic defect.

While the anomalous trichromat uses "anomalous" amounts of primaries for color matches, the dichromat actually *lacks* one kind of cone pigment. The protanope has a loss of red-sensitive pigment, the deuteranope a loss of green-sensitive pigment, and the tritanope a loss of blue-sensitive pigment. Dichromats also see all colors as washed out and desaturated when compared to normal.

A monochromat requires only one of the three primaries to match an unknown. Monochromats suffer from achromatopsia ("without color"), which is distinguished in two forms, rod monochromatism and cone monochromatism.

In rod monochromatism, the person is born with no functioning cones in the retina. These patients have poor visual acuity, absent color vision, nystagmus, photophobia, and an absent flicker response on electroretinography (ERG) testing.

Cone monochromats are very rare. They are totally without the means to discriminate hue. These persons do have cones, but all the cones contain the same visual pigment. (Physiologically, at least two kinds of cones are required to discriminate colors.) These patients have no color sense at all, but do have normal visual acuity, normal ERG flicker response, and no nystagmus (unlike the rod monochromat).

Decrease in color vision can be genetic (congenital) or indicative of pathology (acquired). The pseudoisochromatic plates (Ishihara color plates [Kanehara Trading Inc, Toyko, Japan]) are the most commonly used test for congenital color blindness of the red/green deficiency type. However, test results showing a decrease in only one eye are more indicative of retina and optic nerve disease, since inherited disease affects both eyes. Transmission disorders of the optic nerve, such as in optic neuritis, greatly affect color vision sensitivity. Macular disease can also decrease the ability to discriminate color accurately, but will usually cause other symptoms (such as metamorphopsia).

The Bipolar Layer

The bipolar layer is the middle layer of neural transmission and acts as the connecting cable between the photoreceptors and the ganglion layer. It contains several types of cell bodies that have specific functions:

- bipolar cells—the main transmitters from the rods and cones to the ganglion cell layer
- amacrine and horizontal cells—these help integrate all the circuits (think of them as the coordinating team for the bipolars)
- Müller cells—these cells structurally support the retina; they also supply nutrients.

Cystoid macula edema (CME) is a disorder in which there is cystic swelling of the macula in these inner layers of the retina. In fluorescein angiography, there is pooling of dye in these cystic spaces, yielding a hyperfluorescence in the affected macular area.

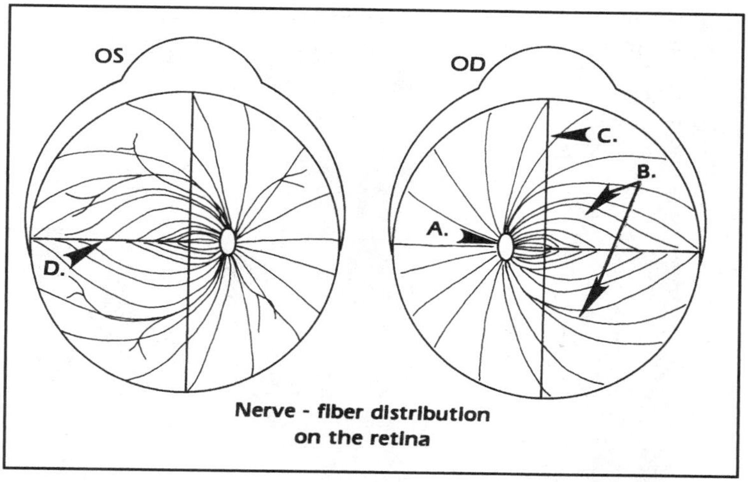

Figure 9-6. Nerve fiber distribution in the retina. (A) Optic disk. (B) Nasal fibers. (C) Vertical meridian. (D) Horizontal raphe. (Courtesy of Norma Garber, Productivity Enhancement Group, Inc.)

The Ganglion Cell Layer

The ganglion cell layer represents the last neural connection for the nerve impulse. The ganglion cells have axons that uniquely pattern together to form the nerve fiber layer (NFL). These axons, or nerve fibers, are the "cables" that converge at the optic nerve head to form the optic disk. They are all part of the optic nerve itself.

The axons of some nerve cells in the body are surrounded by a sheath that aids in the conduction of impulses. The axons of the NFL normally do not have a sheath. When sheathing does appear on the nerve fibers in the fundus, it looks like white patches radiating out from the disk. These are known as medullated or myelinated nerve fibers. These fibers are a normal variant and do not affect visual acuity; however, visual field defects are caused if the myelinated fibers block from reaching any photoreceptors.

Knowledge of the distinctive universal pattern of the NFL (Figure 9-6) is critical to understanding visual field defects. Fibers in the nasal retina go directly to the disk in a radial pattern. Fibers in the temporal inferior retina begin at the horizontal raphe, form an inferior arcuate curve around the macula, and enter the inferior pole of the disk. Fibers in the temporal superior retina begin at the horizontal raphe, form a superior arcuate curve around the macula, and enter the superior pole of the disk. Because of this unique layout, visual field defects directly correspond to the area where the NFL is damaged.

Retinal Vasculature

The retina has two different blood supply networks (Figure 9-7). All retinal vessels are impermeable to fluorescein dye, and therefore any leakage from the vessels constitutes an abnormality.

The Central Retinal Artery and Vein

As a branch of the ophthalmic artery, the central retinal artery (CRA) supplies the inner two-thirds of the retina. It nourishes both the ganglion cells and the bipolar cells. The CRA divides into four main branches at the optic disk: the inferior and superior nasal branches and the inferior and superior temporal branches. If the CRA becomes blocked by debris in the blood stream, the blood supply to the tissues is cut off. A central retinal artery occlusion (CRAO) represents a true

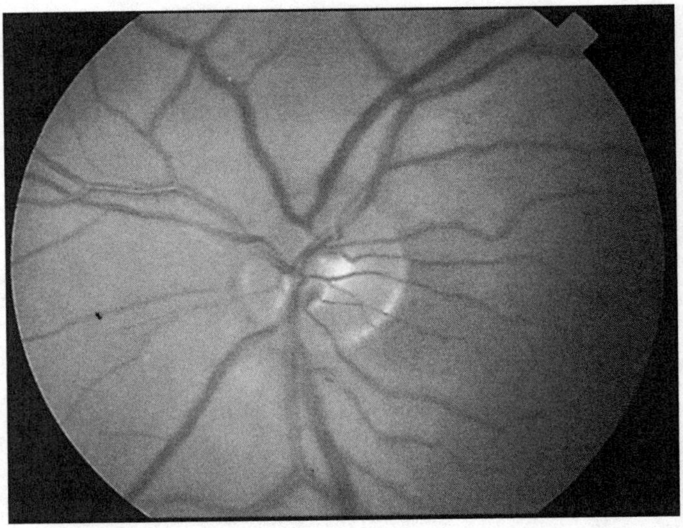

Figure 9-7. Blood vessels of the retina.

ocular emergency, as severe visual loss occurs very rapidly without recovery. Intervention must be immediate before tissue death (due to lack of oxygen) occurs.

The central retinal vein (CRV) also divides in a pattern similar to the CRA. The CRV or its branches can also become occluded (known as a central retinal vein occlusion [CRVO]). In this case, the blockage prevents blood from draining out of the eye. As a result, the veins become engorged. Hemorrhages may occur as pressure builds inside the vessels.

The Choriocapillaris

The outer one-third of the retina (the RPE, rods, and cones) is nourished by the choroid, the highly vascular posterior third of the uveal system. The choroid divides into small capillaries under the scleral surface and forms a fine lobular network called the choriocapillaris.

In approximately 20% of normal eyes, a vessel appearing to be of retinal origin will light up in the prearterial phase of a fluorescein angiogram. This is indicative of a cilioretinal vessel, a vessel of choroidal origin that supplies the macular area, preventing acute central visual loss if the CRA becomes occluded. (In other words, it is a nice extra to have!)

The fovea has a zone surrounding it that is free of capillaries, known as the foveal avascular zone (FAZ). Anatomically in the FAZ there are no vessels or NFL to hinder light processing, giving this area the sharpest vision possible. In fluorescein angiography, there should be no appearance of dye within this zone, and any leakage or staining of dye here indicates a macular disorder.

The Optic Nerve

The optic nerve is the critical circuit connecting the retina with the visual pathway structures. The term for the optic nerve as it appears in the posterior fundus is *optic disk* (also spelled disc), or *optic nerve head*. Another term for the optic disk is *papilla*. In Latin, this means "little mound." The area just surrounding the disk can be described as "peripapillary" (around the disk). The optic disk lies 3 mm nasal to the macula (Figure 9-8). The actual diameter of the disk is approximately 1.5 mm. Often, this dimension will be utilized to describe the location or size of a lesion in the posterior pole. (Example: "nevus approximately 2 disk diameters inferior to the macula.")

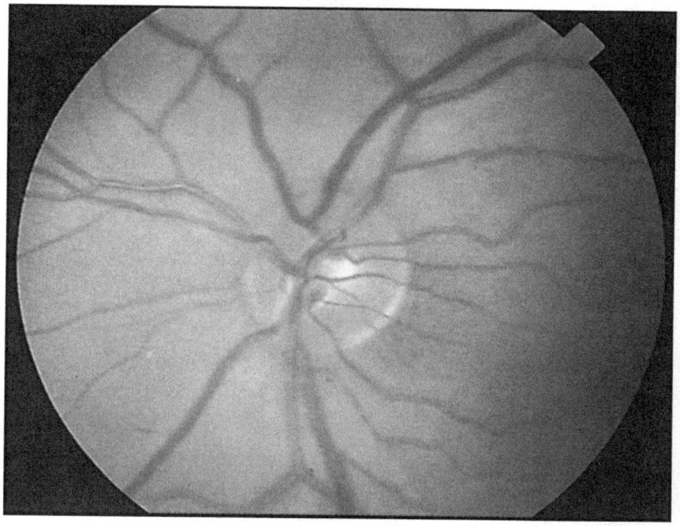

Figure 9-8. Photograph of fundus.

The normal disk has a pink tone because of its supportive vascular system. Pallor, or loss of this pink tone (a whiter looking disk), signifies the loss of a good vascular system. Optic atrophy implies a decrease in the number of nerve fibers. With optic atrophy, there is a definite pallor of the optic disk. There are many causes of optic atrophy, including trauma, toxicity, and pressure on the optic nerve (tumor). The most common cause of optic atrophy is glaucoma. Optic atrophy due to glaucoma is associated with an increased cup size (see next section), whereas other types of optic atrophy are associated more with pallor changes alone.

On a horizontal plane, the disk lies slightly above the true horizontal meridian. This causes the optic disk to be projected somewhat inferior to the horizontal plane in a visual field. The disk extends 5.5 degrees horizontally and 7.5 degrees vertically on a visual field chart. The disk represents an absolute physiologic blind spot in the field of vision. This is because there are no photoreceptors (rods and cones) at this area to photochemically produce impulses. The blind spot is approximately 15 degrees temporal to the macula in a visual field.

The CRA and CRV branch out at the "mouth" of the disk. Both the CRA and CRV exit the disk on the nasal side. The CRA lies nasal to the CRV and often exhibits a "stem" that sends out inferior and superior branches. Generally, the CRA has smaller caliber vessels than the CRV, along with vessels that appear bright red when compared to the purple-red CRV vessels. Both the CRA and CRV form four branches, the inferior and superior temporal branches. While these important vessels pass through the disk, they do not supply it. (The optic disk is nourished by branches of the short posterior ciliary arteries that form a circular arrangement known as the circle of Zinn.)

The Optic Cup

The optic disk has a normal depression, or physiologic cup, in its center from the recession of fetal tissue. The color of the cup is whiter than the rest of the disk. This cup varies greatly in size from one individual to another. The cup size of the disk is an important measurement because various disease processes can affect it. This measurement is known as the cup to disk ratio (C/D ratio) (Figure 9-9). This ratio is first assessed as a fraction—the disk representing a "10," and the proportion of the cup representing a percentage of that overall "10." For example, if a cup is

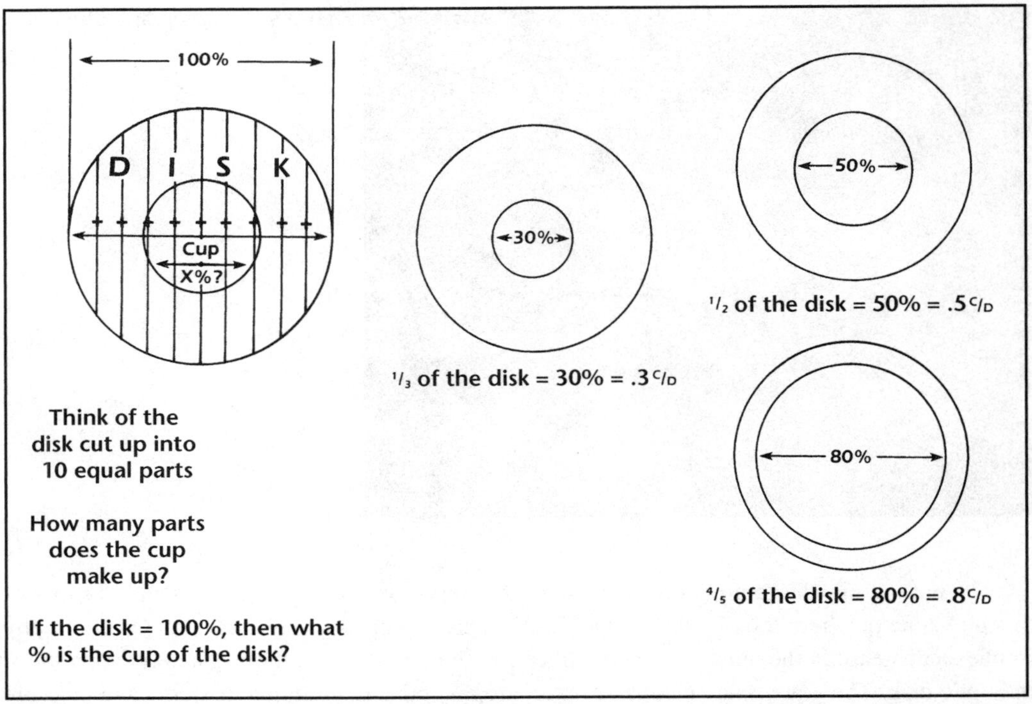
100%
D I S K
Cup
X%?
Think of the disk cut up into 10 equal parts
How many parts does the cup make up?
If the disk = 100%, then what % is the cup of the disk?
30%
1/3 of the disk = 30% = .3 C/D
50%
1/2 of the disk = 50% = .5 C/D
80%
4/5 of the disk = 80% = .8 C/D

Figure 9-9. C/D estimation technique. (Reprinted with permission from Nemeth SC, Shea CA. *Medical Sciences for the Ophthalmic Assistant.* Thorofare, NJ: SLACK Incorporated; 1988.)

assessed at 5/10 of the overall diameter of the disk, that C/D ratio equals 0.5. If a cup is assessed at 8/10 of the overall diameter, the C/D ratio is 0.8. As a general rule, the normal C/D ratio is 0.3.

The lamina cribrosa is the sieve-like membrane that is sometimes visible at the posterior extension of the cup. The nerve fibers pass through this lamina and lie in the small canals of the sieve as they pass through. Visually, the lamina cribrosa appears like a pocket of microfine holes in the bottom of the cup. It can be more apparent in the pathologic cupping of advanced glaucoma (Figures 9-10 and 9-11).

A normal cup has a "rim" of tissue surrounding it. The rim is composed of the nerve fibers entering the conduit. Think of a healthy rim as a tire fully inflated with air. When damage occurs to this rim (as with increased IOP), the tire, or rim, begins to thin or "notch" out.

The Glaucomatous Disk

Optic disk evaluation is a critical part of a basic ocular examination. Careful assessment of the optic nerve head is the most sensitive method of detecting pathological changes in the early stages of glaucoma. Currently, studies are suggesting that structural damage to the optic nerve can be apparent before visual field loss is documented.

The areas of the optic nerve head most susceptible to early increased IOP are the superior and inferior poles of the disk. The fibers entering here are from the temporal retina and arch around the macula. Destruction of temporal fibers will cause visual field deficits that mirror the exact "cable pattern": arcuate nasal scotomas and nasal steps. (See the Basic Bookshelf title *Visual Fields* for details of glaucomatous field testing techniques.) Because glaucoma causes damage to these fibers as they converge on the nerve head, there is a gradual "erosion" and loss of mass as

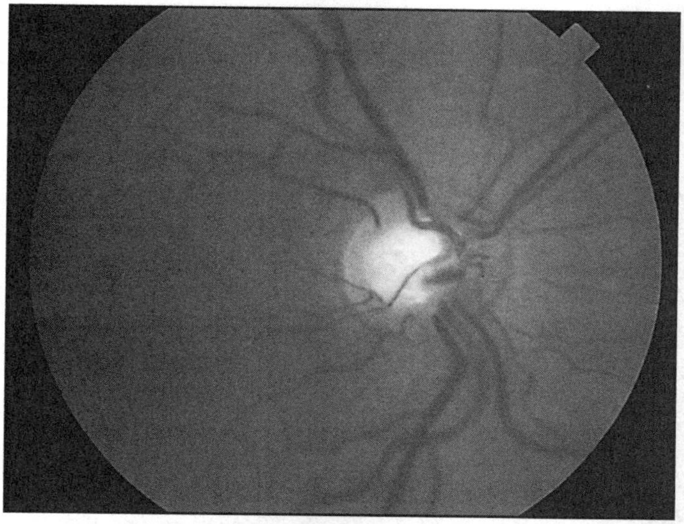

Figure 9-10. Increased C/D ratio as seen in glaucoma.

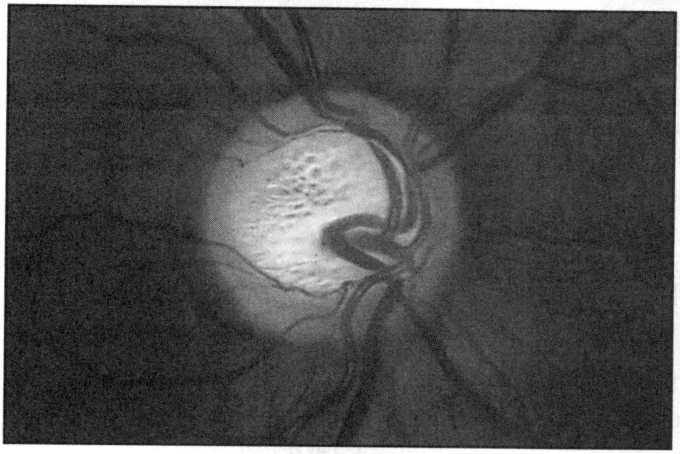

Figure 9-11. Close-up of cupping.

the fibers die. This loss of fibers at the nerve head causes an increase in the total amount of cupping (or a decrease in the neural rim tissue). A progressive increase in cup size is diagnostic of glaucoma (Figure 9-12).

There are other clinical signs that help separate the C/D ratio in glaucoma from other disease processes. The changes significant of glaucoma are as follows:

- asymmetry of cup size between the eyes
- enlargement of the cup primarily in the vertical axis, or pole
- notching, or small dug out area of the disk
- pallor, or whiteness, of the nerve head (especially temporally)

The Myopic/Hyperopic Disk

In high degrees of myopia, the axial length (AL) of the eye is increased. Consequently, the nerve often enters the globe obliquely, causing some traction and pulling on the temporal side. This pulling causes the retinal pigment layer to be pulled away and the sclera to be exposed temporally, revealing a whitish crescent called the temporal crescent (Figure 9-13). Sometimes

Figure 9-12. Progression of optic cupping in glaucoma. (Reprinted with permission from Nemeth SC, Shea CA. *Medical Sciences for the Ophthalmic Assistant.* Thorofare, NJ: SLACK Incorporated; 1988.)

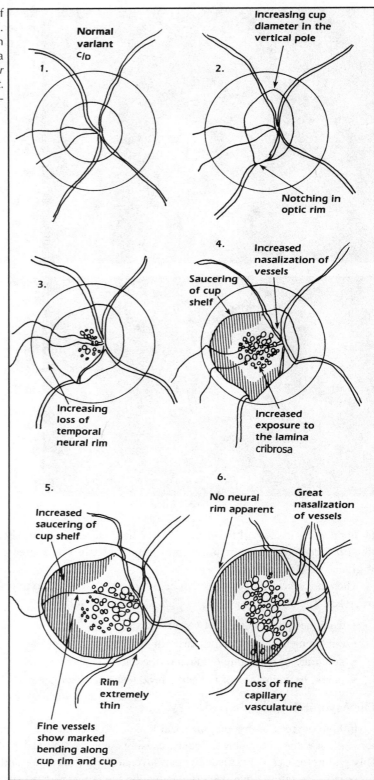

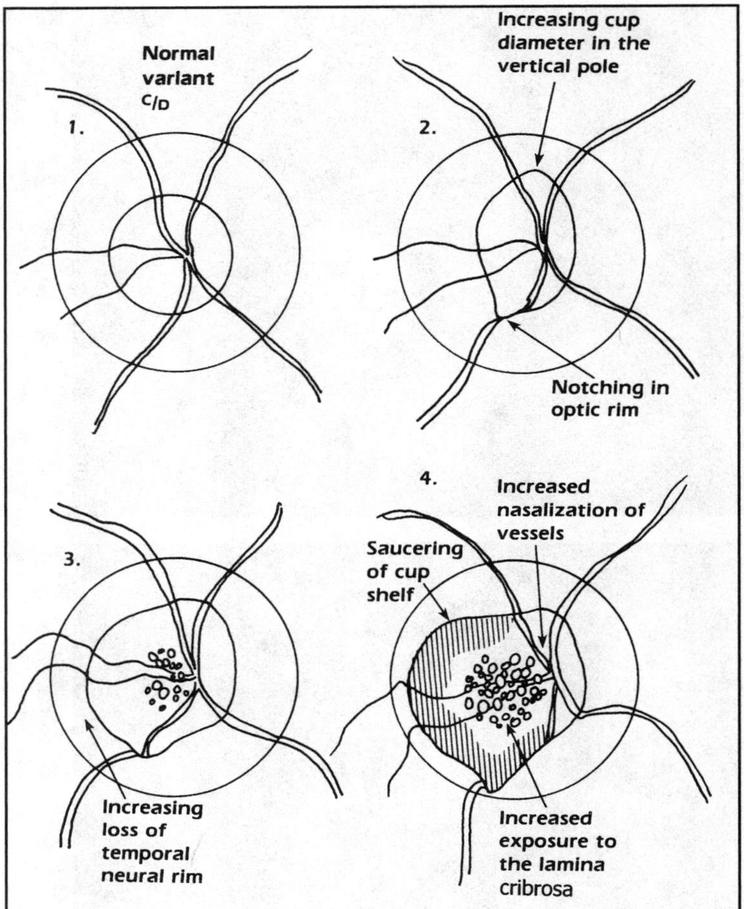

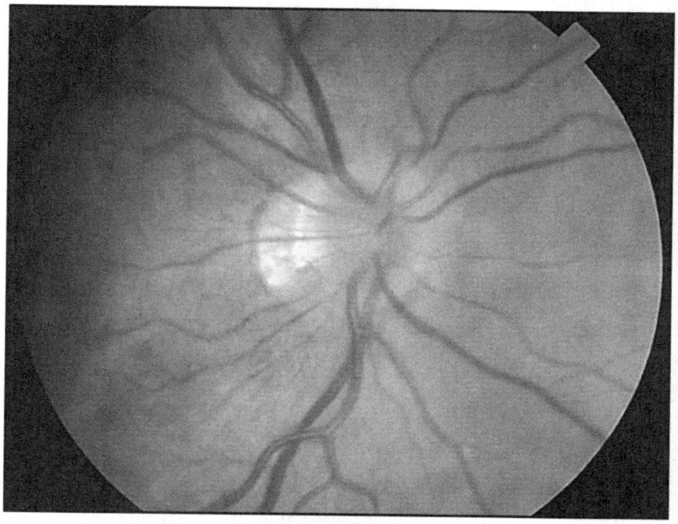

Figure 9-13. Temporal crescent in a myopic eye.

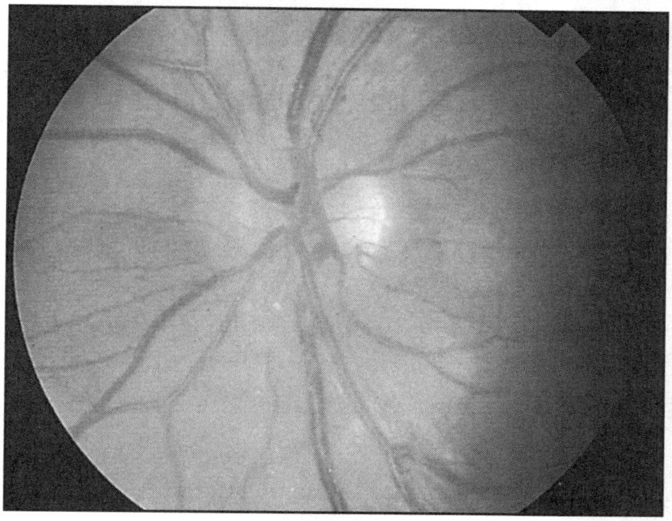

Figure 9-14. Hyperopic disk.

pigment will fill in the crescent, and it will be black. This is a normal variant. In general, myopes have higher C/D ratios than emmetropes. On visual field examination, myopes with larger C/D ratios can exhibit slightly enlarged blind spots.

The C/D ratio in the hyperope is generally less than the emmetrope, and often the cup is actually absent (Figure 9-14). This is due to the crowding of the nerve fibers into a smaller scleral opening than normal. Consequently, hyperopic disks can have the appearance of a pseudopapilledema (the false appearance of a swollen optic nerve).

Evaluation of the Retina, Macula, and Optic Disk

Evaluation of Function

Clinically, there are many tests we perform just to test the well-being of the macula and its foveal peak. *Visual acuity testing* is essentially a test of macular function, as well as the tests described next. (For specific how-to's for many of these tests, please consult the Basic

Bookshelf titles *Clinical Skills for the Ophthalmic Examination: Basic Skills* and *Special Skills and Techniques*.)

Potential acuity meter (PAM)—This is designed to project an eye chart onto the retina in such a way so as not to be affected by media opacities like cataracts or corneal disease. It gives an estimation of potential macular function when acuity is reduced from these media opacities (as opposed to true macular disease). The PAM mounts on a slit lamp and has an adjustment to compensate for the patient's spherical refractive error.

Laser interferometer—This creates an interference pattern from two out-of-phase light waves and projects it onto the retina. The resulting image appears as numerous parallel lines that can be adjusted from large to small. The patient is asked to identify the smallest lines he or she can resolve. This device will penetrate even very dense media opacities that may hinder the PAM, but its diagnostic intent is basically the same (ie, to evaluate macular function without intervening media opacities).

Entopic phenomena—In some situations where the retina cannot be visualized, detecting the presence of entopic phenomena can be a very useful and rapid test of macular function. This test involves creating an image of the patient's own retinal vessels by rapidly moving a light back and forth next to the eye. When patients can appreciate this image (and compare it to a good eye), it may offer information about potential macular function.

There are different kinds of *color vision tests* that vary in their mode of operation, the defects they detect, their sensitivity and ability to quantify errors, and their ease of administration.

- *Pseudoisochromatic plates*—These are the most common screening tests for color vision, among them being the well-known Ishihara plates and the American Optical H-R-R plates (American Optical, Southbridge, MA). The plates are composed of a figure (often a number) of colored dots in a background of different colored dots. A person with a color defect does not see the figure or may see a different figure than a normal person would. The Ishihara plates detect very subtle red/green defects only, while the American Optical H-R-R plates detect red/green and blue/yellow defects. These plates were designed to identify patients with x-linked congenital color defects, the most common of the color defects.
- *Farnsworth Panel D-15*—This is a test of color discrimination ability using an arrangement design. The patient arranges a set of colored caps according to their similarity. The D-15 test evaluates color confusion and will only detect severe anomalous trichromatopsia and dichromatopsia. It is fairly rapid to administer and easy for patients (even children) to comprehend.
- *Farnsworth-Munsell 100 hue test*—This is a very detailed arrangement test that has 84 colored caps varying in hue but with constant lightness and saturation. After the patient arranges these caps in a natural color order, the score is calculated and displayed on a graph. Both congenital and acquired color defects have definitive patterns on this detailed test. Deuteranopes, protanopes, and tritanopes (as well as achromats) have very distinguishable patterns on the graph. This test is very tedious and time-consuming to administer, and yet it is extremely sensitive and lends itself to a high degree of quantification.
- *Nagel anomaloscope*—This test's mode of operation is the matching of luminosity. Luminosity losses in the spectrum range from subtle (in the anomalous trichromat) to very pronounced (in the monochromat). The anomaloscope allows the patient to match spectral yellow to a red/green mixture by varying the brightness of the yellow test field. It detects only red/green defects and requires a fairly high degree of patient cooperation.

Contrast sensitivity testing (CST)—CST has been suggested as a method to analyze patients for very early decreases in contrast awareness, which can be an indicator of NFL death. Contrast sensitivity is derived by measuring the lowest detectable contrast across a wide range of spatial frequencies. Contrast sensitivity and visual acuity are correlated in a normal patient (ie, reduced acuity secondary to refractive errors has a known effect on contrast sensitivity). Diseases such as optic neuritis, glaucoma, diabetic retinopathy, and amblyopia are known to cause decreased contrast sensitivity with near-normal visual acuity.

Visual field testing—Evaluation of the visual field via perimetry and other techniques is yet another method of retinal evaluation. Retinal visual field defects (posterior to the ganglion and NFL) are rather unique in that most of the pathology causing the defect is quite visible with the ophthalmoscope or by using contrast dye, such as fluorescein angiography. The field defects are opposite to the location of the lesion in the retina, as a lesion found in the temporal retina will project a defect in the nasal visual field. Defects at the retinal level can be irregular and can cross the vertical or horizontal meridian. They are always monocular, as opposed to the binocular patterns of chiasmal and postchiasmal disease (see Chapter 10). Macular disease can result in a 5 degree central scotoma and can be clinically correlated with poor visual acuity and color vision. (Macular disease can be bilateral, but usually there is asymmetry in the scotoma size and depth of defect. Clinical correlation is always needed.)

Other retinal pathologies causing visual field defects include retinitis pigmentosa (mid-peripheral ring scotomas or true gun-barrel fields), RDs (sharp peripheral, usually quadrantal, constriction unilaterally in the affected eye), and choroiditis (asymmetric defects, often unilateral, with no respect to the horizontal or vertical meridian).

The NFL death caused by increased IOP in glaucoma leads to decreased sensitivity of the retina. This is well-documented by performing a visual field exam, which will generally show a decrease in the decibel value on the actual value scale of the printout. It also results in an increase in the difference in decibel response to the age-related norm. (See the Basic Bookshelf title *Visual Fields.*)

Amsler grid—This is a sensitive visual field test that can detect early changes within the macula (ie, the central 10 degrees of the visual field). It is a grid of small boxes with a dot in the center (as a fixation point). In macular disease, the patient may see distortions, wavy lines, or sometimes missing lines. This distortion is termed *metamorphopsia* (change of form). Often, patients with macular disease will complain that newspaper print looks like "scrambled eggs" or "trying to read while looking through water." This distortion is the result of the photoreceptors in the retina becoming disturbed and "tilted" by disease processes. The Amsler grid is often used as a home-testing device to monitor and follow types of macular diseases.

Electro-oculography (EOG)—The function of the RPE layer is objectively measured by EOG. This is an electrical recording test based on the standing potential of the eye. Metaphorically, the eyeball acts like a battery with a measurable voltage between the cornea and back of the globe. This measurable voltage is referred to as the standing, or resting, potential of the eye. EOG is a measure of RPE-photoreceptor complex. Electrodes are placed on either side of the eye and the patient watches an alternating target, moving the eyes side to side. The voltage changes are translated into pen movement on a polygraph. As the eye moves between two fixed points, this movement is translated into an electrical change. EOG is a tedious and lengthy test, both for the patient and the operator. EOG primarily aids in the diagnosis of Best's disease, otherwise known as vitelliruptive macular dystrophy. The normal "light rise" is absent in patients with this disease. Even carriers of this disease with no fundus changes show an abnormal EOG light rise.

Electroretinography—ERG is usually used as a complementary test with EOG. ERG is an objective electrophysiology test that evaluates the retina's response to light. Contact lens-type electrodes are placed on the cornea. The patient is exposed to both scotopic and photopic light stimulations, and results are electrically recorded and graphically displayed on a computer. The A-wave generated from this response is primarily produced by the photoreceptor cells, while the B-wave is a response from the bipolar cells. Retinitis pigmentosa classically produces an abnormal or extinguished ERG (depending on the stage of the disease), as it is a rod-cone dystrophy. A classic example of a disease in which the EOG is abnormal but ERG is normal is Best's disease, a primary macular dystrophy that begins in childhood.

Evaluation by Visualization

Direct visualization of the fundus is possible via *ophthalmoscopy.* Direct ophthalmoscopy gives a magnified view (15X) of the nerve head and allows for a rapid assessment of the neural elements of the disk, even through an undilated pupil. The instrument has a variety of both plus and minus internal lenses to aid in the examination of eyes with refractive errors or for viewing objects anterior to the retinal plane. The field of view is limited to about 6.5 degrees. As it is a monocular instrument, there is no stereopsis and consequently subtle contour changes can be missed. *Indirect* ophthalmoscopy consists of a light source and binocular viewing device worn around the forehead like a miner's headlight. The light is focused through the (dilated) pupil by a condensing lens (ie, +20 diopters) and the retinal image is inverted by the plus optics of the patient's eye and the condensing lens. The wide-angle inverted image has stereoscopic detail that is actually exaggerated. While all of the retina can be examined, this device is most useful for peripheral retinal exams.

The fundus can also be examined at the *slit lamp* with a small *90 diopter lens*. Excellent stereopsis can be achieved, but pupil dilation is often necessary. In addition, *ophthalmic endoscopy* can be used during surgery to visualize the retina.

Fundus photography is used to provide a permanent record of retinal entities. *Stereo fundus photography* involves photographing the optic nerve by taking images from slightly disparate angles. This gives the examiner an excellent study of the nerve with a high degree of both stereo and magnification. Documentation of the nerve's appearance on each patient visit allows for a visual comparison to watch for clues of a progressing disease.

B-scan ultrasonography (ultrasound)—This allows for indirect visualization of the vitreous and retina when there is a poor or absent view of the posterior segment secondary to trauma, cataracts, or any anterior segment disruption. For example, by using different amounts of sensitivity, the B-scan can help the clinician differentiate between a simple vitreous hemorrhage and a vitreous hemorrhage with a RD. Tumors or elevations of the retinal plane can also be photographically documented and quantified.

Fluorescein angiography (FA)—This provides dynamic information about the retinal and choroidal circulation as well as the status of the RPE. Pathologic changes can be detected in each of these layers by studying a time sequence of photographic images taken as dye initially transits, and subsequently recirculates, during the study period. Clinically, the FA is frequently used in assessing diabetic macular edema and/or ischemia, as well as in the search for subretinal neovascular membrane (SRNVM) in suspected wet ARMD.

Innovations in Imaging of the Retina and Optic Nerve Head

The past decade has seen technology evolve into clinical instruments of diagnostic value, especially for posterior segment anatomy. The rapid improvements of this technology even within a few years' time is on a continuum with even more excitement ahead. This section is a short introduction to imaging technologies that are either currently available in the marketplace or are evolving into future clinical devices.

Optical Coherence Tomography

Optical coherence tomography (OCT) is based on the physical principle of imaging reflected light of the posterior segment while resolving depth. The beam of light is from 800 to 1400 nm wavelength in the near infrared. This technology has allowed remarkable cross-sectional views of tissue (ie, the retina) that appear similar to that seen under a microscope. OCT has opened up a new universe for clinically correlating a flat two-dimensional world (ie, traditional fundus photography) with that of a three-dimensional visualization of retinal pathology.

Perhaps the simplest way to understand OCT is to compare it to the A-scan. A-scan is clinically used for measuring the AL of an eye from anterior cornea to anterior retina. OCT is actually composed of many A-scans of the 10-layered retina. The amplitude of reflection (measured in decibels) is plotted against tissue depth.

The OTC scans a 3.2-mm diameter circle surrounding the nerve head. A graph of the superior, nasal, inferior, and temporal NFL thickness values is given in a shaded area on the exam printout for a normal value, and the individually scanned NFL thickness plotted within the normal range. A NFL color-coded map is generated, with yellows and reds representing thicker areas (normally superior and inferior sectors) and greens and blues representing thinner areas (normally nasal and temporal sectors) (Figure 9-15).

Scanning Laser Tomography or Confocal Scanning Laser Ophthalmoscope

Currently, the main clinical application of the scanning laser tomography (SLT) is the evaluation of the optic nerve head in three-dimensions. The SLT employs a 675-nm, near infrared diode laser to collect reflected light at various depths of laser focus. The instrument produces cross-sectional images along the axial plane (or z-axis) of the optic nerve head. A confocal pinhole is used for filtering light that is not from the exact focal plane of the desired target. Each pixel is assigned a reflectometry measurement along the z-axis, and a reflectivity image is produced. Maximum reflectivity is assumed to be the height of the location in space, and from this data a topographic image is generated.

The stereometric optic nerve head parameters are generated for six designated sectors surrounding the optic nerve head (ie, temporal, temporal/superior, temporal/inferior, nasal, nasal/superior, and nasal/inferior), some of which include the rim area, the C/D ratio, and an average retinal NFL thickness. The latest generation uses a relevance vector machine and generates statistical probability of glaucoma using ethnic-specific databases.

Scanning Laser Polarimetry

Scanning laser polarimetry (SLP) uses a polarimeter and a confocal scanning laser ophthalmoscope to quantitatively measure the NFL. When polarized light passes through the NFL, the birefringent (bends or refracts light in two different directions) nature of this tissue causes two polarized components to be produced. The slower axis is aligned with the axon arrangement, while the difference in light propagation in the opposite axis produces a retardation (ie, slowing down) that is in proportion to the NFL thickness.

Retinal Thickness Analyzer

The retinal thickness analyzer (RTA) is a computerized biomicroscopic system that employs a green HeNe laser as a slit beam to produce an optical cross-section of the retina and disk. Sixteen optical cross sections 200 μm apart are imaged over a 3 mm × 3 mm area. This is done rapidly

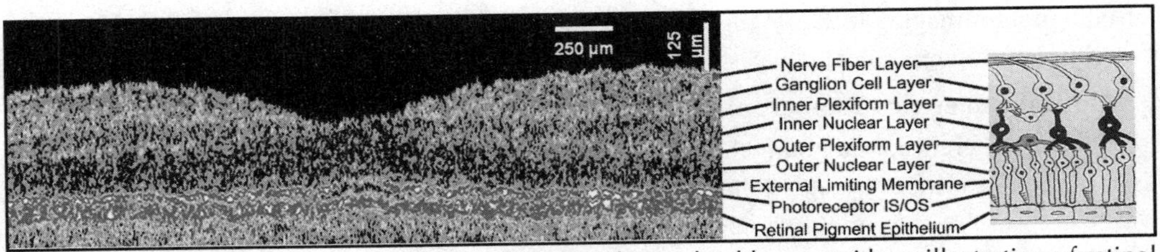

Figure 9-15. A comparison of a macular OCT image from a healthy eye with an illustration of retinal morphology. The print out is actually color-coded for easier interpretation. (Reprinted with permission from Schuman JS, Puliafito CA, Fujimoto JG. *Everyday OCT: A Handbook for Clinicians and Technicians*. Thorofare, NJ: SLACK Incorporated; 2007.)

(330 msec) to eliminate eye movement artifacts. A two- or three-dimensional map of retinal thickness is generated by an automatic algorithm.

The RTA was the first device used to study the evolution of macular holes. The RTA is also used for objective measurement of retinal thickness to evaluate for clinically significant macular edema before and after focal laser treatment. An understanding of macular thickening via quantitative devices such as the RTA will help in developing thresholds for drug treatment therapies at certain stages of disorders such as diabetic macular edema.

Ocular Blood Flow Imaging

The vascular anatomy of the eye is quite complex. The retinal vascular system and uveal system are both supplied by the ophthalmic artery via the retrobulbar vessels. Disorders of clinical significance include glaucomatous optic neuropathy, diabetic retinopathy, and (in some theories) ARMD.

Color Doppler imaging (CDI) is a B-scan ultrasound application that produces blood velocity measurements using pulsed Doppler. The operator applies the B-scan probe in a similar manner as performing a B-scan of the globe. The peak systolic velocities and end-diastolic velocities in the retrobulbar blood vessels can be calculated once the peak and trough of the wave are identified by the operator.

Some instruments use FA and ICG to quantitate blood flow. Fluorescein dye in conjunction with the SLO may be used to measure blood flow dynamics such as the arteriovenous passage time and mean dye velocity.

Glossary of Common Disorders

age related macular degeneration (ARMD): Deterioration and death of the photoreceptors in the macular region of the retina with consequential degrees of loss of central vision; two subtypes of ARMD have been classified: "dry," or nonexudative, is the most common. "Wet," or exudative, is the more severe type, causing extreme visual loss as abnormal blood vessels bleed beneath the retina.

angioid streaks: Tiny breaks in Bruch's membrane that look like linear "cracks" in the retina; associated with degeneration of elastic fibers of the body.

anomalous trichromat: Abnormality or deficiency of one of the three primary pigments (red, green, or blue) of the retinal cones. This is the most common type of "color blindness."

asteroid hyalosis: "Snowball-like" opacities composed of calcium soap deposits in the vitreous humor; is usually a result of aging, occurs unilaterally, and does not affect vision.

branch retinal vein occlusion (BRVO): Obstruction of one branch of the main retinal vein; visual loss is dependent on how much of the macula has been affected.

central retinal artery occlusion (CRAO): Acute and sudden blockage of the central retinal artery (usually from a blood clot) with a painless vision loss; frequently causes irreversible vision loss up to blindness. On ophthalmoscopy, the retina appears pale and the macula frequently has a "cherry red spot" appearance.

central retinal vein occlusion (CRVO): Blockage of the central retinal vein from a clot that can cause visual loss. On ophthalmoscopy, the retina appears congested with large areas of flame hemorrhages.

chorioretinitis: Inflammation of the choroid and retina.

cystoid macular edema (CME): Swelling of the macula as a result of disease, injury, or eye surgery. Fluid collects within the layers of the macula, causing blurred and distorted central vision. Macular edema that occurs with diabetic retinopathy is termed *diabetic macular edema (DME)*. Clinically significant macula edema (CSME) is treated with small focal laser spots to alleviate the fluid and restore visual acuity.

drusen: Whitish or yellowish deposits in the retina; one of the hallmark early signs in age-related macular degeneration. Drusen occur at the level of Bruch's membrane and have been classified according to their shape, size, and edge appearance (ie, hard, soft, and soft indistinct).

endophthalmitis: Severe inflammation of the tissues of the internal structures of the eye; causes include bacterial infection following postoperative intraocular surgery and retained intraocular foreign bodies. Endophthalmitis can be visually devastating.

flashes/floaters: Flashes appear as "lightening streaks" to the subject and occur when the vitreous tugs on the retinal surface (*see* vitreous detachment). Floaters are generally cell debris that drifts through the vitreous cavity and casts a shadow on the retina; they can appear as spots, "bugs," "cobwebs," or hairs. While flashes and/or floaters are usually benign, they can be the hallmarks of a RD.

metamorphopsia: Distortion of visual images; frequent symptom in age-related macular degeneration (especially the "wet" type); commonly detected via Amsler grid.

optic atrophy: Wasting away of the optic disk resulting from degeneration of the nerve fibers of the optic nerve, most commonly caused by glaucoma.

pallor: Pale or increased white appearance; in ophthalmology used to describe the tone of the rim of the optic nerve head. Optic nerve pallor is one of the characteristics of glaucoma.

papilledema: Swelling, congestion, and elevation of the optic nerve head secondary to increased intracranial pressure.

pseudopapilledema: Literally, "false papilledema"; the optic nerve head appears swollen but this is actually a normal variant (usually seen in patients with high degrees of hyperopia).

retinal detachment (RD): A pulling away of the retina from the posterior scleral surface of the eye; common causes include trauma, high myopia, and advanced diabetic retinopathy.

retinitis*: General term referring to inflammation of the retina.

retinitis pigmentosa*: Inherited retinal dystrophy in which deposits of melanin pigment appear on the retina, accompanied by atrophy of retinal blood vessels and pallor of the optic disk, eventually leading to loss of vision.

subretinal neovascular membrane (SRNVM; also called choroidal neovascular membrane): Condition in which a crack in Bruch's membrane allows vessels from the choroidal circulation to grow into the space beneath the retina. These fragile vessels leak fluid and/or blood, leading to severe loss of central vision. The most common condition associated with a SRNVM is "wet" ARMD.

synchysis scintillans: A degenerative vitreous condition in which cholesterol crystals accumulate in the vitreous cavity; they appear as small white floaters suspended in the posterior segment.

syneresis: Degeneration of the vitreous, usually with age, as the vitreous humor loses its gel-like composition and becomes more fluid.

temporal crescent: A whitish semi-circle on the temporal aspect of the optic disc; this is a normal variant more frequently seen in myopes.

uveitis: Inflammation of the uvea, the vascular tunic of the eye. Anterior uveitis is inflammation specific to the anterior segment of the eye (also called iritis), while posterior uveitis is specific to the posterior segment. Panuveitis refers to a general, wide-spread uveal inflammation.

vitreous detachment: Separation of vitreous humor from the retina, most commonly occurring in the periphery.

vitreous hemorrhage: Bleeding into the vitreous humor that may be removed surgically via vitrectomy. In diabetics, this most commonly happens from abnormal, fragile blood vessels in the advanced stages of proliferative diabetic retinopathy.

vitritis: Inflammation of the vitreous humor secondary to infection, autoimmune disorders, and (in rare instances) tumors. Symptoms may include spots and/or sensitivity to light.

window defect: A specific focal type of hyperfluorescence seen on retinal fluorescein angiography where the fluorescein is visible due to loss of a small focal area of the retinal pigment epithelium layer.

* These definitions are used with permission from Ledford JK, Hoffman J. *Quick Reference Dictionary of Eyecare Terminology, Fifth Edition.* Thorofare, NJ: SLACK Incorporated; 2008.

Chapter 10

Visual Pathway

Al Lens, COMT

KEY POINTS

- Understanding the anatomy and physiology of the visual pathway aids in localizing lesions.
- Lesions located in front of the chiasm (prechiasmal) will affect only one eye; lesions at or behind the chiasm will affect both eyes.
- The eyes only collect the images that we see. The brain is responsible for interpreting what is viewed.
- Conditions such as dyslexia are caused by poor interpretation of what is viewed.
- Various parts of the brain respond to visual stimuli. The response ranges from recognizing the image to sending impulses to other parts of the body to respond to what has been seen.
- Important terms to remember when relating to visual field include:

    congruous—similar defect in each eye

    hemianopsia—defect in right or left half of visual field, usually right and left

    homonymous—relating to the same half of each eye's visual field

    incongruous—defect(s) lacks similarity in each eye

    quadrantanopsia—defect in one quarter of the visual field

Anatomy

The human visual pathway consists of the optic nerves, optic chiasm, optic tracts, lateral geniculate nuclei, optic radiations, and the visual cortex (Figure 10-1). Although the visual pathway ends here, the visual system also involves other parts of the brain for image recognition, interpretation, eye movement coordination, and motor response.

The photoreceptors within the retina are stimulated by light entering the eye. Each receptor converts the information into an electrochemical signal. Transmitters carry this signal to bipolar cells in the retina's middle layer (see Chapter 9). These cells send the information to the ganglion cells in the innermost layer of the retina. From here, the signal enters axons, which lead to the optic nerve.

The optic nerve is also referred to as cranial nerve number two (CN II). As it leaves the eye, the optic nerve passes through the lamina cribrosa. The length of the optic nerve is sufficient to provide some slack; this permits eye movement without producing tension on the nerve. After leaving the globe, the optic nerve is encased in a myelin sheath. At the apex of the orbit, the nerve runs through the circle of Zinn—a ring of fibrous tissue that constitutes the origin of most of the extraocular muscles (EOMs). The optic nerve then enters the optic canal. After exiting the canal, the nerve passes through the rigid outer membrane of the brain (the dura mater).

As the retinal fibers leave the eye, the peripheral fibers are located peripherally in the optic nerve. The macular fibers occupy a temporal sector of the nerve. As the optic nerve approaches the optic chiasm, the macular fibers tend to spread out and intermix across the diameter of the nerve. The temporal fibers stay in the temporal aspect of the nerve, and the nasal fibers are positioned nasally in the nerve.

The two optic nerves (one from each eye) join together above the pituitary gland. This junction forms the optic chiasm where the nasal fibers from each eye cross and join the temporal fibers of the fellow eye. Most fibers that cross at the chiasm are from the macula, which predominate inferiorly at this juncture in the visual pathway. Some of the crossed fibers loop a short distance into the optic nerve of the fellow eye, creating the knee of von Willebrandt.

The nasal fibers are responsible for the temporal visual field. As a result of the crossover that occurs at the optic chiasm, the fibers responsible for the visual field to the right of the midline travel along the left side of the brain, and vice versa. The crossing of half of the fibers plays an important role in stereo vision (see Chapter 14).

Upon exiting the optic chiasm, the newly joined nasal and temporal fibers form the right and left optic tracts. Immediately posterior to the optic chiasm, the tracts are cylindrical in shape. They become more flattened as the distance from the chiasm increases. The upper temporal fibers move to a medial position and the lower temporal fibers are in the inferior lateral position. Upper nasal fibers are seen in the inferior-medial position in the optic tract, while the lower nasal fibers occupy the lateral aspect of the optic tract.

The optic tract enters the lateral geniculate body, which is an elevation produced mostly by the lateral geniculate nucleus. It is here that the retinal fibers from each eye are organized into matched pairs and synapse with visual neurons. Other sense organs also send information to the lateral geniculate body. Some scientists believe the lateral geniculate bodies are responsible for shutting out visual input to the brain when attention is given to other sensory input.

The optic radiation (geniculocalcarine pathway) is composed of axons from the lateral geniculate cells and carries the visual impulses to the occipital lobe. The axons from the superior portion of the lateral geniculate body proceed directly to the occipital visual cortex. Inferior axons form Meyer's loop as they extend around the lateral ventricle (a cavity containing

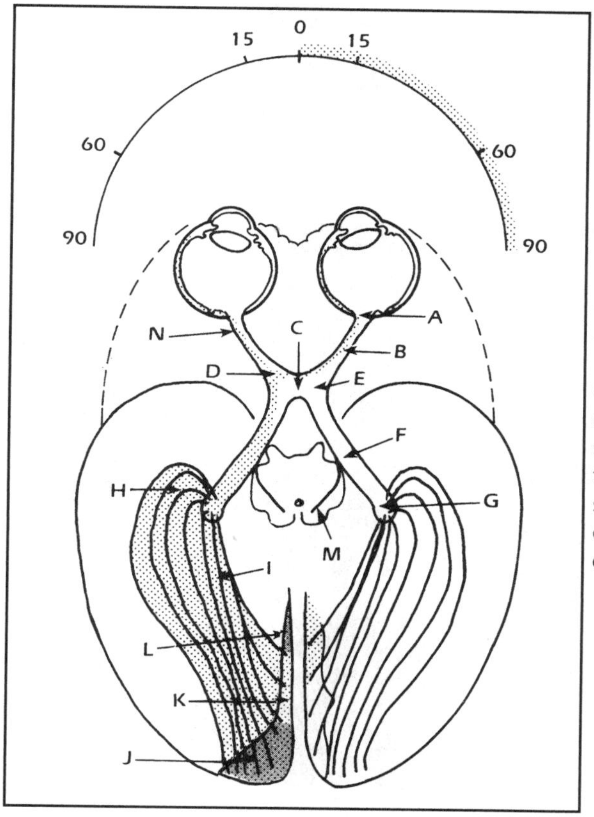

Figure 10-1. Visual pathways. (A) The optic nerve. (B) The nasal retinal fibers in the optic nerve. (C) Nasal fibers crossing at the chiasm. (D) Von Willebrandt's knee of the right eye's nasal fibers positioned in the left optic nerve. (E) Chiasm or crossing. (F) The optic tract. (G) The lateral geniculate body. (H) Meyer's loop of the temporal radiations. (I) Parietal optic radiations. (J) Macular area of the calcarine cortex in the occipital lobe. (K) Peripheral binocular calcarine cortex. (L) Monocular (extreme peripheral) calcarine cortex. (M) Afferent fibers to the brainstem which are comprised of about 10% of the visual sensory information. (N) Temporal fibers from the retina traveling on the same side of the head to the same side visual cortex. (Courtesy of Norma Garber, Productivity Enhancement Group, Inc.)

cerebrospinal fluid) on their way to the visual cortex. There are three main groups of fibers in the optic radiations. The superior portion contains the fibers for the superior aspect of the retina (serving the inferior visual field). Conversely, the inferior fibers of the optic radiations serve the superior visual field. The central field, or macular area, has its fibers in the central portion of the optic radiations.

The primary visual cortex is also known as the striate cortex or Brodmann area 17. It is located along the calcarine fissure in the occipital lobe. The visual impulses are received in this area, and the image is finally "seen." The visual cortex is surrounded by a visual association area that interprets the visual information so the brain can recognize what is being viewed.

Physiology

When the anatomy of the visual pathway is completely understood, localizing visual field defects is relatively simple. The chiasm plays an important role in locating the cause of visual field defects (Figure 10-2). Prechiasmal lesions (those in the retina or optic nerve) will be isolated to the affected eye. Chiasmal lesions cause bitemporal defects (ie, in the temporal field of both eyes). Postchiasmal lesions will affect both eyes, but on the opposite side of the visual field (ie, a lesion in the left visual pathway will result in a right visual field defect). The more congruous, or similar, the defect is in each eye, the farther back in the pathway the lesion occurs. Be aware, however, that defects encountered in the clinic often do not match what is depicted in textbooks. This is especially true for mild defects, as examples in books often demonstrate extreme cases.

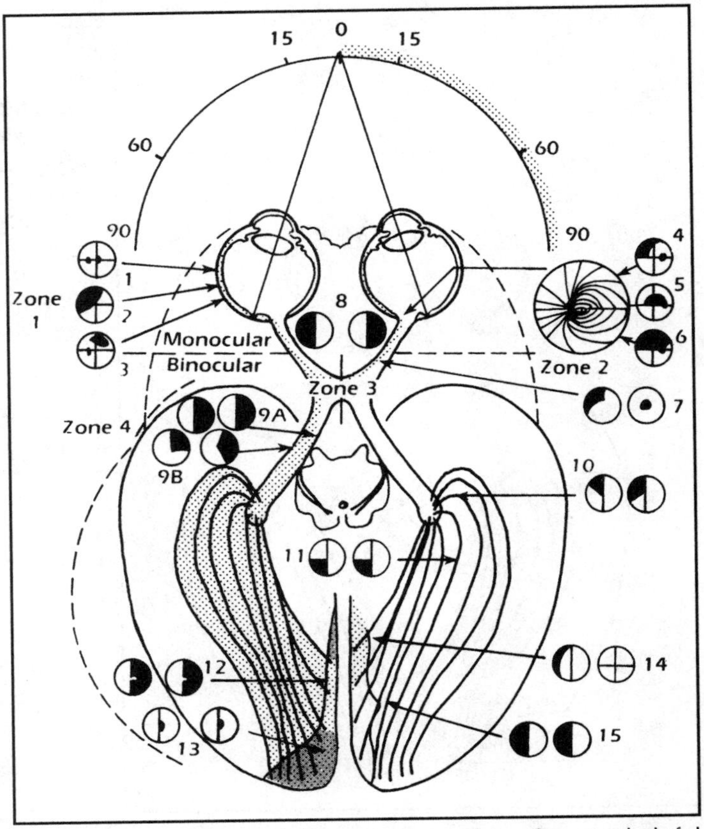

Figure 10-2. Typical field patterns seen with damage along the visual pathways. **Zone 1**—Retinal: 1. central scotoma; 2. RD; 3. isolated scotoma. **Zone 2**—The NFL: 4. nasal step; 5. arcuate scotoma; 6. altitudinal radiating scotoma. **Zone 3**—The chiasm: 7. prechiasmal anterior junctional scotoma; 8. chiasmal bitemporal hemianopsia. **Zone 4**—The retrochiasmal regions: 9A. optic tract complete right homonymous hemianopsia; 9B. optic tract incomplete incongruous hemianopsia; 10. temporal lobe left incongruous quandrantanopsia; 11. parietal lobe left congruous quandrantanopsia; 12. macular sparing occipital homonymous hemianopsia; 13. congruous occipital right macular hemianopsia; 14. left temporal crescent damage to deep right occipital cortex; 15. left complete homonymous hemianopsia. (*Note:* Complete homonymous hemianopsias can occur anywhere posterior to the chiasm. If they are incomplete, they are helpful in localizing pathology. As a general rule, the more anterior the pathology, the more unlike or incongruous the field defects. The more posterior the pathology, the more exquisitely congruous the field defects become.) (Courtesy of Norma Garber, Productivity Enhancement Group, Inc.)

Light travels in a straight line. For example, light coming from an object in the temporal visual field will pass through the cornea on a relatively straight path to the nasal retina. (It is not possible for the light to bend dramatically and end up on the temporal retina. Therefore, light from the inferior-temporal visual field will fall on the superior-nasal retina.) It makes sense, then, that retinal lesions will cause a defect in the exact *opposite* quadrant of the visual field. A lesion in the superior-nasal retina will cause an inferior-temporal visual field defect, for example.

As the nerve fibers leave the eye via the optic nerve, they travel in a location similar to that of their origin (ie, fibers from the superior-nasal retina are located in the upper-nasal portion of the optic nerve). Therefore, lesions on the optic nerve will produce a visual field defect in the *same* quadrant as the lesion.

As previously discussed, the nasal fibers cross over at the optic chiasm to join the temporal fibers of the fellow eye. Since the nasal fibers are responsible for the temporal visual field, it is understandable that a lesion in this area would cause a field defect affecting the temporal field of both eyes (bitemporal). The vertical midline in the visual field would be respected (the defect will not extend beyond the midline), so the defect would be referred to as a hemianopsia (a defect in the right or left half of the visual field). The most common cause of an optic chiasm lesion is a tumor in the pituitary gland, which lies just beneath the chiasm.

The optic tract is composed of nasal retinal fibers from one eye and the temporal retinal fibers from the other eye. Since association of these newly joined fibers occurs later in the visual pathway, a lesion in the optic tract will cause a homonymous defect (on the same side of the visual field) but will usually be incongruous (dissimilar). Lesions in the left optic tract will cause a right visual field defect in both eyes, or more technically, a right homonymous visual field defect.

The lateral geniculate body is the site of matching for the fibers from each eye. A lesion in this area would typically cause a congruous, homonymous hemianopsia. However, since other input from other senses is received in this area, it is quite possible to have a visual field defect with other sensory symptoms. In fact, it is often the presence of other sensory loss that will implicate the lateral geniculate body rather than the optic radiations (which would produce similar visual field defects).

The optic radiations that represent the superior quadrants of the retina advance almost straight back to the visual cortex. A lesion in the parietal lobe would affect these fibers, causing an inferior visual field defect. (Remember that the superior retina is responsible for the inferior visual field.) The inferior quadrants of the retina are served by the lateral fibers in the optic radiations that loop forward (Meyer's loop). A superior visual field defect would be caused by a lesion in this area. Homonymous right field defects are caused by lesions in the left visual pathway.

The visual cortex is the termination of the optic radiation fibers. The macular region occupies a large portion of the posterior visual cortex. The superior quadrants of the retina terminate on the superior portion of the calcarine fissure, while the fibers for the inferior quadrants terminate inferiorly. Lesions in this area will usually produce congruous defects (matching in both eyes). Retention of the central 5 degrees (macular sparing) is not uncommon with visual cortex lesions.

The visual pathway is only the beginning of a very complex visual system. The brain must not be forgotten when considering vision. In fact, the eyes are often considered to be merely extensions of the brain. While all of the anatomic structures required for vision are present at birth, the brain must learn how to see. Studies have been done in which kittens were placed in environments lined with vertical or horizontal stripes, but not both. After several months, the kitten that was in the room with vertical stripes was unable to detect horizontal surfaces. The other kitten, having seen only horizontal lines, walked into chair legs and other vertical objects. The visual portion of the human brain is fully developed by 6 to 10 years of age. Failure to have clear vision by this age will result in permanently decreased vision, even after the cause of the visual impairment is treated. This type of arrested visual development is known as amblyopia.

Dyslexia is a condition in which the brain misinterprets the written word. It is believed that the left hemisphere of the brain functions differently in dyslexics than in normal individuals. Dyslexia causes problems translating language to thought or thought to language. It also causes problems with reading and writing and difficulty decoding (reading) and encoding (spelling) words, resulting in impaired reading comprehension, as well as difficulties in mathematics, usually relating to sequencing of steps or directionality. Since dyslexia is an anatomical defect in the brain, it is not possible to "grow out" of it, nor is it an ocular problem. However, people with dyslexia are often very intelligent and creative despite their impaired ability to read—Albert Einstein and Thomas Edison are thought to have been dyslexic.

Glossary of Common Disorders

Bjerrum's area: Arc-shaped area of the visual field extending from the optic nerve to the nasal horizontal meridian.

congruent (also called congruous): Similarity of size and location of visual field defects in each eye.

hemianopsia (also called hemianopia): Visual field defect affecting one half of the visual field, typically the nasal or temporal halves. May also be altitudinal (defect of the upper or lower half of the visual field).

homonymous: Visual field defect that exists on the same side (right or left) in each eye.

incongruent (also called incongruous): Visual field defect in one eye lacks similarity to that of the other eye (mainly in size and shape).

nasal step: Visual field defect with decreased sensitivity beginning 20 to 30 degrees nasal to fixation; a difference in the upper and lower defects gives the defect a step-like appearance at the horizontal midline of the visual field; typically indicates the presence of glaucoma.

quadrantanopsia (also called quadrantanopia): Visual field defect affecting one quadrant of the visual field in each eye.

scotoma (also called blind spot): Area within the visual field that has an abnormal decrease or loss of sensitivity.

Chapter 11

Nerve Supply

Al Lens, COMT

KEY POINTS

- The human body has 12 pairs of (CNs) that originate in the brain.
- Remembering the order of the cranial nerves is made easier by using a mnemonic: *O*h, *o*h, *o*h, *t*o *t*ouch *a*nd *f*eel *v*ery *g*ood *v*elvet, *ah*. (Olfactory, optic, oculomotor, trochlear, trigeminal, abducens, facial, vestibulocochlear [acoustic], glossopharyngeal, vagus, accessory [spinal accessory], and hypoglossal.)
- All CNs that have a motor function also have proprioceptors—receptors that respond to stimuli such as pressure, position, or stretching. This is a feedback mechanism so the brain is aware of posture, movement, and changes in equilibrium, as well as knowledge of position, weight, and resistance of objects in relation to the body.
- Seven of the 12 pairs of CNs are associated with the eye: CNs II through VIII.
- The vestibular system is interconnected with the oculomotor system. This allows the head to be rotated while keeping the eyes fixated on an image.

The nervous system is a network of delicate nerve cells interlaced with each other. It consists of two divisions, the central (brain and spinal cord) and peripheral nervous systems (sensory, cranial, and spinal nerves with their branches to the entire body). This chapter will cover the peripheral nerve supply to the eye and its tissues.

The peripheral system can be broken into two divisions, one for incoming data (afferent) and one for outgoing responses (efferent). The efferent division consists of the autonomic (involuntary) system, which governs involuntary processes such as heart beat and visceral action, and the somatic (voluntary) system which controls skeletal muscles (including the intraocular muscles).

The autonomic system itself has two branches: the sympathetic and parasympathetic. The sympathetic division is stimulated by stress, causing the "fight or flight" reactions of rapid heartbeat, increased breathing rate, sweating, pupil dilation, and decrease in the energy spent on visceral activities. The parasympathetic branch regulates the normal, resting-state tasks of digestion and other bodily functions.

The nervous system is a network of delicate nerve cells interlaced with each other. It consists of two divisions, the central (brain and spinal cord) and peripheral nervous systems (sensory, cranial, and spinal nerves with their branches to the entire body). This chapter will cover the peripheral nerve supply to the eye and its tissues.

The peripheral system can be broken into two divisions, one for incoming data (afferent) and one for outgoing responses (efferent). The efferent division consists of the autonomic (involuntary) system, which governs involuntary processes such as heart beat and visceral action, and the somatic (voluntary) system which controls skeletal muscles (including the intraocular muscles).

The autonomic system itself has two branches: the sympathetic and parasympathetic. The sympathetic division is stimulated by stress, causing the "fight or flight" reactions of rapid heartbeat, increased breathing rate, sweating, pupil dilation, and decrease in the energy spent on visceral activities. The parasympathetic branch regulates the normal, resting-state tasks of digestion and other bodily functions.

Cranial Nerves

The body has 12 pairs of CNs that are part of the peripheral nervous system (Table 11-1 and Figure 11-1). As the word *cranial* implies, these nerves have their origin in the brain. Each CN is named, usually according to the most important structure it innervates or to its primary function. The CNs are also numbered according to their site of origin, anterior to posterior. The first two pairs originate from the forebrain and the rest originate from the brainstem. They all serve only head and neck structures except the vagus nerves, which extend into the ventral body cavity.

Those nerves that send their impulse to the brain are called sensory nerves. Motor nerves send impulses from the brain to muscles. Some CNs are both sensory and motor (mixed functions).

The olfactory nerve (CN I) originates from the nasal cavity and synapses in the olfactory bulb. The fibers of the olfactory bulb form the olfactory tract, which terminates in the olfactory cortex. CN I is responsible for the sense of smell. (Damage to this nerve can cause a loss of smell.)

The optic nerve (CN II) originates from the retina of the eye, extending to the optic chiasm where the nasal fibers from each retina cross over to join the temporal fibers of the fellow eye. This leads to the optic tract, which synapses in the lateral geniculate body. This gives rise to the optic radiations which extend to the occipital cortex. CN II is a purely sensory nerve, responsible for vision. (Damage to the optic nerve can cause loss of sight.)

Table 11-1
Cranial Nerves

CN #	Name	Motor/Sensory	Function
I	Olfactory	Sensory	Smell
II	Optic	Sensory	Sight
III	Oculomotor	Motor	Movement of eye (MR, SR, IR, and IO), pupil constriction, accomodation, and upper lid elevation
IV	Trochlear	Motor	Superior oblique muscle
V	Trigeminal	Mixed	Sensation of touch in face, nose, forehead, temple, tongue, and eye. Innervation for chewing.
VI	Abducens	Motor	Lateral rectus muscle
VII	Facial	Mixed	Reflex tearing, facial expression, some taste, and blinking
VIII	Vestibulocochlear (acoustic nerve)	Sensory	Hearing and equilibrium
IX	Glossopharyngeal	Mixed	Taste and swallowing
X	Vagus	Mixed	Taste, heart rate, breathing, digestion, and voice
XI	Spinal Accessory	Motor	Innervation of neck and shoulder muscles, provides posture and rotation of head
XII	Hypoglossal	Motor	Tongue movement

The oculomotor nerve (CN III) originates from the ventral midbrain and passes through the superior orbital fissure on its way to the eye. CN III innervates three of the four rectus muscles (superior, inferior, and medial) and the inferior oblique muscle. Other muscles innervated by CN III are the levator palpebrae superioris (upper eyelid elevation), iris sphincter (pupil constriction), and ciliary muscle (accommodation). (Damage to CN III can cause double vision as the eyes drift outward. Loss of accommodation and ptosis can also occur with CN III damage.)

The trochlear nerve (CN IV) originates from the dorsal midbrain and enters the orbit (along with CN III) through the superior orbital fissure. This nerve is responsible for the superior oblique muscle. This innervation can be easily remembered by noting that the superior oblique muscle runs through the trochlea. (Damage to CN IV can cause double vision and loss of ability to rotate the eye down and in.)

The trigeminal nerve (CN V) originates from the pons (a mass of nerve cells on the surface of the brainstem) to the face. CN V has three divisions: ophthalmic, maxillary, and mandibular. The ophthalmic division is responsible for sensation from the scalp, nose, nasal cavity, cornea, upper eyelid, and lacrimal gland. The maxillary division carries impulses from the nasal cavity, mouth, upper lip, and lower eyelid. The mandibular division is distributed to the tongue (excluding taste buds), lower teeth, and skin of the temples and chin; it also innervates muscles for chewing. (Damage to CN V can cause intense pain or a loss of sensation in the aforementioned areas, as well as difficulty chewing.)

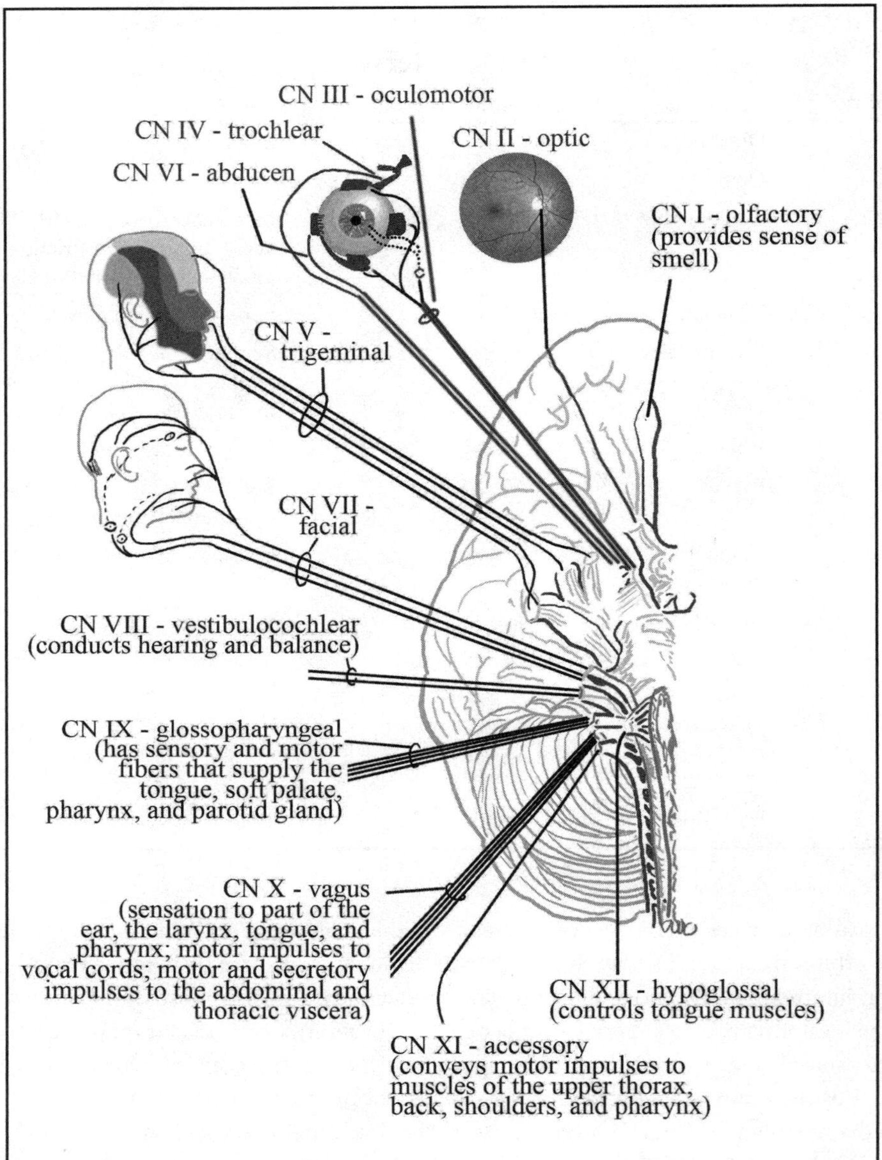

Figure 11-1. Cranial nerves and their functions.

The abducens nerve (CN VI) originates from the inferior pons and, like CNs III and IV, enters the orbit through the superior orbital fissure. The lateral rectus muscle is innervated by CN VI. (Damage to this nerve will cause limitation of abduction, and esotropia may be noted.)

The facial nerve (CN VII) originates adjacent to CN VI in the pons and is distributed throughout the ear, face, palate, and tongue. There are five major branches: temporal, zygomatic, buccal, mandibular, and cervical. The facial nerve is responsible for facial expression; taste from the anterior two-thirds of the tongue; and autonomic (involuntary) impulses to the lacrimal, nasal, and palatine glands and the sublingual and submandibular salivary glands. (Damage to CN VII can cause paralysis of the muscles on one side of the face, which can result in the inability to close the eye, wrinkle the forehead, or whistle. The mouth will appear deviated *away* from the affected side.)

The vestibulocochlear (acoustic) nerve (CN VIII) originates at the junction of the pons and the medulla, then passes through the internal auditory meatus to enter the inner ear. This nerve consists of two divisions: vestibular and cochlear. Vestibular relates to the middle part of the inner ear that is behind the cochlea and in front of the semicircular canals. Cochlear relates to a winding cone-shaped tube that forms another portion of the inner ear, adjoining the vestibule. The vestibulocochlear nerve is responsible for hearing and equilibrium. (Damage to CN VIII can result in deafness or dizziness, loss of balance, and nausea.)

The glossopharyngeal nerve (CN IX) originates from the medulla. It then distributes to the pharynx (tube connecting the mouth to the esophagus), ear, meninges, posterior third of tongue, and parotid (salivary) gland. CN IX has six branches: carotid, tympanic, pharyngeal, lingual, tonsillar, and the sinus nerve of Hering. The glossopharyngeal nerve plays a role in taste, swallowing, gag reflex, salivation, and blood pressure regulation. (Damage to this nerve can cause impaired taste and problems in swallowing.)

The vagus (pneumogastric) nerve (CN X) originates from the medulla and extends into the neck, thorax, and abdomen. This nerve has the widest distribution of all the CNs. CN X plays a role in speech, digestion, heart rate, taste, and breathing. (Damage to CN X can cause loss of voice, difficulty in swallowing, and impaired digestion. Total destruction of this nerve would cause death.)

The accessory nerve (CN XI) is made up of two segments, spinal and cranial. The spinal portion emerges from the superior region of the spinal cord and joins with the cranial root that originates from the medulla (located just above the spinal cord). The union is only temporary before they diverge to neck (cranial division) and shoulder (spinal division) regions. The cranial division joins the vagus nerve, adding its motor and some of its cardioinhibitory fibers. The spinal division is responsible for head and neck movement. (Damage to this nerve will cause drooping of the shoulder and an inability to rotate the head away from the affected side.)

The hypoglossal nerve (CN XII) originates from the medulla with distribution to the extrinsic and intrinsic muscles of the tongue. (Extrinsic muscles are those outside the tongue that control its position. Intrinsic muscles are inside the tongue and control its movement.) CN XII contributes to speech, swallowing, and mixing of food during chewing. (Damage to one of these nerves can result in paralysis of one side of the tongue, thick speech, and deviation of the tongue toward the affected side.)

Innervation of Extraocular Muscles

As detailed previously, the six pairs of extraocular muscles (EOMs) responsible for eye movement are innervated by three pairs of CNs: III, IV, and VI. Many people use the simulated formula $(LR_6SO_4)^3$ to remember what muscle is innervated by which nerve. This mnemonic means that the lateral rectus muscle is innervated by the sixth CN (LR_6), the superior oblique's innervation is from the fourth CN (SO_4), and all other muscles receive their innervation from the third CN (^{3}).

The nerves are appropriately named: oculomotor, trochlear, and abducens nerves for CNs III, IV, and VI, respectively. Since four of the six muscles are innervated by CN III, it is fitting that it is named the oculomotor nerve. The superior oblique muscle travels through the trochlea (pulley) and is innervated by the trochlear nerve (CN IV). Lastly, the lateral rectus muscle, which is responsible for abduction, is innervated by the abducens nerve (remember: ABDuction/ABDucens). In addition to innervating the EOMs, these nerves also send messages to and from the ciliary body, iris sphincter, and levator superioris.

Eye movements can hold a gaze steady, counteract head movement, or shift the gaze to look at a new object. As one muscle receives innervation, its yoke muscle (contralateral synergist, or paired muscle in fellow eye) receives equal innervation to move the eyes together in parallel. This is known as Hering's law.

Sherrington's law indicates that when one EOM receives an impulse to contract, its opposing muscle (antagonist) in the same eye receives an impulse to relax an equal amount.

Sympathetic and Parasympathetic Systems

The autonomic nervous system (ANS) is concerned with control of involuntary bodily functions. This includes regulating the function of smooth muscle tissue, the heart, and the glands (especially the gastric, salivary, and sweat glands, as well as the adrenal medulla). It is divided into the sympathetic (thoracolumbar) system and the parasympathetic (craniosacral) system.

The sympathetic system is made up of the ganglionated sympathetic trunk, its connections with the thoracic and lumbar segments of the spinal cord, the large and small splanchnic nerves (distributed to the abdominal organs), and certain ganglia in the abdomen. The sympathetic fibers enter the paravertebral ganglion in the sympathetic trunk after leaving the spinal cord's thoracic and lumbar segments. At this juncture, the preganglionic axons can synapse with a postsynaptic neuron or pass through without synapsing. The latter forms the splanchnic nerves, which synapse with prevertebral ganglia.

Postganglionic fibers from the upper (cervical) region of the sympathetic trunk serve the eye, lacrimal gland, nasal mucosa, submandibular and sublingual glands, parotid gland, and some of the heart.

Stimulating sympathetic fibers usually produces pupillary dilation, vasoconstriction in the part supplied, a general rise in blood pressure, erection of the hairs, sweaty skin, secretion of small quantities of thick saliva, depression of gastrointestinal and urinary tract activity, and acceleration of the heart. These activities occur as part of the "fight or flight" system—a response to stress situations (danger, anger, excitement, etc) that require the expenditure of energy. Norepinephrine is the major transmitter agent of the sympathetic system.

The parasympathetic system includes fibers of some of the CNs (such as the motor fibers of the vagus) and of other fibers connected with the sacral part of the spinal cord. The preganglionic fibers originate from nuclei in the midbrain, medulla, and sacral portion of the spinal cord. They pass through CNs III, VII, IX, and X, as well as the second, third, and fourth sacral nerves. The fibers synapse with postganglionic neurons located in autonomic ganglia in the walls of (or near) the organ innervated.

Preganglionic fibers of the parasympathetic system extend from the central nervous system to the structures to be innervated. They synapse with terminal ganglia inside or close to the target organ, where postganglionic axons complete the transmission. Acetylcholine is the only transmitter agent of the parasympathetic system.

Stimulation of the parasympathetic system produces contraction of the pupil, vasodilation of the part supplied, general fall in the blood pressure, copious secretion of watery saliva, increased gastrointestinal activity, and slowing of the heart. Generally speaking, the parasympathetic system counteracts and is much less complex than the sympathetic system.

Glossary of Common Disorders

Bell's palsy (also called facial palsy, seventh nerve palsy): Temporary condition affecting the left or right seventh (facial) cranial nerve; eye-related symptoms include difficulty or inability to close the eye, lack of tear production, drooping eye brow, drooping lower lid, and sensitivity to light (related to dry eye). Other symptoms can include drooping mouth and lack of control of forehead muscles on the affected side.

CN III (oculomotor) palsy: Paralysis of the third (oculomotor) cranial nerve; affected eye turns down and out, pupil is dilated, and accommodation is decreased or absent. The patient typically reports double vision, increased sensitivity to light, and difficulties with reading (for non-presbyopic patients).

CN IV (trochlear) palsy: Paralysis of the fourth (trochlear) cranial nerve; affected eye is elevated (especially when the patient tries to look down) and rotated outward (causing the patient to tilt the head opposite to the affected side).

CN VI (abducens) palsy: Paralysis of the sixth (abducens) cranial nerve; affected eye turns inward, causing double vision that worsens with distance viewing or when gazing in the direction of the affected side.

nystagmus: Involuntary eye movement caused by instability of the motor sensory system controlling the eyes; can be congenital or acquired.

ocular muscle abnormalities: see Glossary of Common Disorders, Chapter 5.

pupil abnormalities: See Glossary of Common Disorders, Chapter 8.

Chapter 12

Vascular Supply and Lymphatics

Al Lens, COMT

KEY POINTS

- Arteries carry blood away from the heart and always run deep within body tissues.
- Deep veins are paired with like-named arteries. Superficial veins are readily visible in the limbs, face, and neck.
- The cardiovascular system relies on the lymphatic system to return fluid to the bloodstream.
- Lymph nodes act as filters to engulf and destroy pathogens, as well as to trap particulate matter in the lymphatic stream.
- The body's defense against the invasion of foreign substances (antigens) consists of specific and nonspecific mechanisms that join to form the immune system.

Cardiovascular System

The cardiovascular system, consisting of the heart and blood vessels, delivers blood to tissue cells to provide oxygen and nutrients. In exchange, the blood picks up the waste excreted by cells. The heart is a pump that propels blood through miles of blood vessels throughout the body. Arteries are responsible for carrying blood away from the heart, and veins return blood to the heart.

Large conducting arteries take blood to the medium- and smaller-sized distributing arteries. From here, arterioles deliver blood to the tiny capillaries that branch out through most of the body's tissues. Nutrient molecules and blood cells are able to escape from the capillaries, completing the delivery of nutrition and oxygen to the tissues.

In turn, the capillary bed must collect blood to be delivered back to the heart. The venous equivalent of arterioles are called venules. These tiny vessels join to form veins. The blood pressure inside veins is much lower than that of arteries. Valves in the veins, as well as skeletal and respiratory muscle pumps, assist in returning blood to the heart.

In addition to delivering oxygen and nutrients to tissue cells, the flow of blood removes wastes from tissue cells, absorbs nutrients from the digestive tract, allows blood to be processed by the kidneys, and is involved in gas exchange in the lungs. (For more on the cardiovascular system, see the Basic Bookshelf title *General Medical Knowledge for Eyecare Paraprofessionals*.)

Arterial Supply to the Eye

The head and neck receive their blood supply via four paired arteries—common carotid arteries, vertebral arteries, thyrocervical trunks, and costocervical trunks (Figure 12-1). The principal blood supply to the head and neck comes from the carotid arteries. Vertebral arteries serve the posterior head and neck (Figure 12-2). The thyrocervical and costocervical trunks are short vessels that supply blood to the inferior neck.

The common carotid arteries travel through the lateral aspect of the neck then divide to form external and internal carotid arteries, beginning at the superior border of the larynx. The external carotid arteries supply most of the tissues on the outside of the skull. This includes the scalp, face, teeth, lower jaw, chewing muscles, tongue, larynx, nasal and pharyngeal mucosa, thyroid gland, and dura mater.

The internal carotid arteries are the principal blood supply of the cerebrum (largest part of the brain). The ophthalmic artery is the main branch of the internal carotid artery and supplies blood to structures in and around the orbit, as well as to the nasal cavity and anterior scalp. The internal carotid artery then divides into anterior and middle cerebral arteries to serve the medial surface of the cerebral hemisphere and lateral parts of the temporal and parietal lobes, respectively.

The central retinal artery (CRA) branches off the ophthalmic artery near the optic canal (Figure 12-3). The path of the CRA takes it beneath the optic nerve until it pierces the dura and arachnoid 10 to 15 mm behind the eye. After a short distance, it bends toward the center of the nerve. As the artery enters the eye, it travels up the nasal side of the cup of the optic disk. Here it forms two branches called the inferior and superior branch arteries (Figure 12-4). (Refer to Chapter 9 for more detail on retinal vasculature.)

Carotid artery insufficiency can cause amaurosis fugax (sudden, transient loss of vision) by temporarily decreasing the blood supply to the eye. Assessing arterial insufficiency can be done using numerous methods, including *palpation* of the carotid arteries in the neck or *angiogram* of the carotid system. Measuring the ophthalmic artery pressure can be done using *ophthalmodynamometry*—pressure is applied to the globe using the dynamometer, and the diastolic reading is recorded from the instrument when pulsation of the retinal arterioles is seen. Systolic pressure is determined when the pressure is increased until the first complete collapse of retinal arterioles is seen.

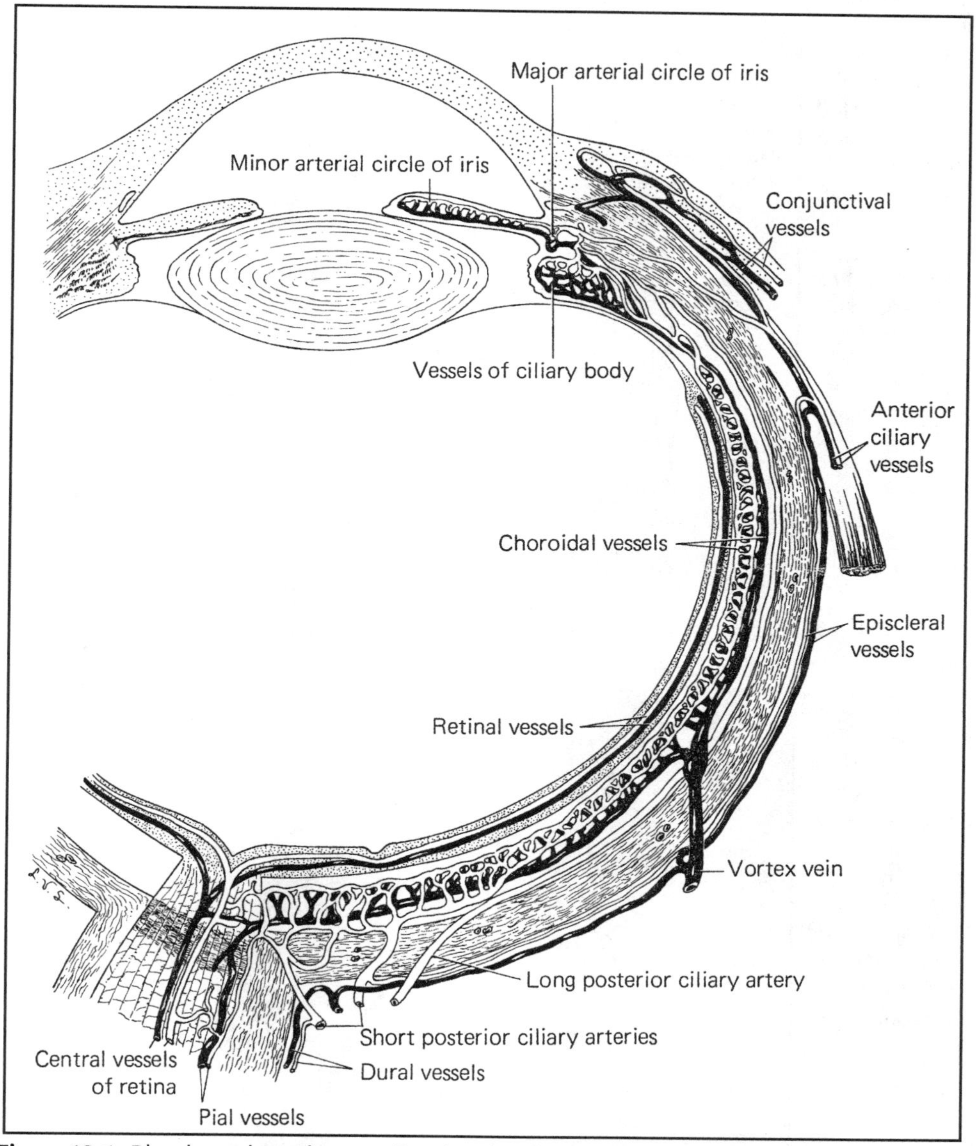

Figure 12-1. Blood supply to the eye. (Reprinted with permission from Vaughan DG, Asbury T, Riordan-Eva P. *General Ophthalmology.* 13th ed. Norwalk, CT: Appleton and Lange; 1992.)

The posterior and anterior ciliary arteries deliver blood to the ciliary body. Blood vessels in the iris originate from the major arterial circle in the ciliary body. The normal cornea, like the lens, is avascular (has no blood vessels). Therefore, nutrition for these structures must come from a source other than the blood, such as the aqueous humor. The tear film also provides nourishment to the cornea.

The conjunctiva and anterior episclera receive their blood supply from the palpebral and anterior ciliary arteries, which stem from the ophthalmic artery. The posterior episclera derives its blood supply from the long and short posterior ciliary arteries, which also arise from the ophthalmic artery. The sclera is relatively avascular and is supplied by the vasculature of the episclera and choroid.

Figure 12-2. Blood supply on the surface of the brain. (Reprinted with permission from Cassin B, ed. *Fundamentals for Ophthalmic Technical Personnel.* Philadelphia, PA: WB Saunders; 1995.)

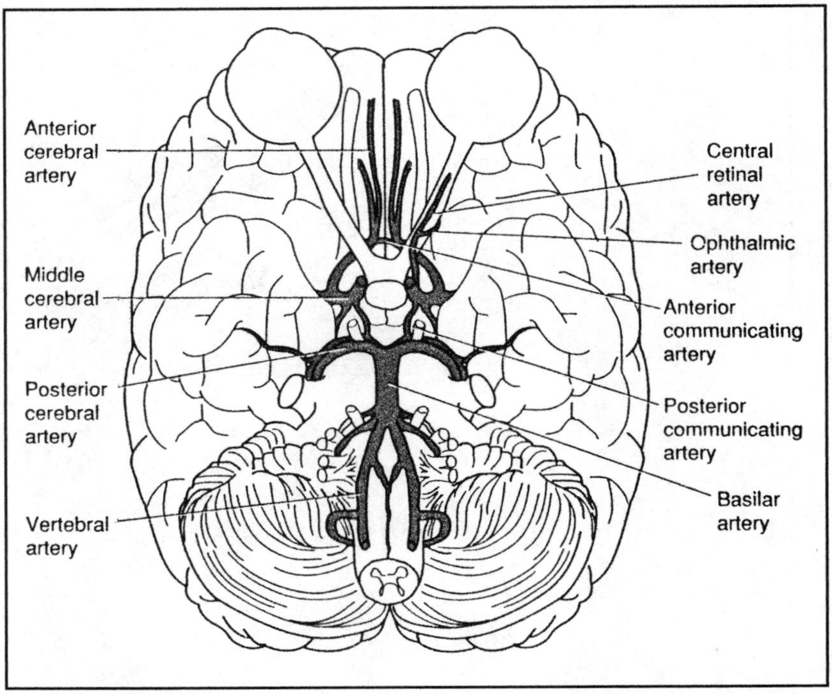

Figure 12-3. Ophthalmic artery and its branches. (Reprinted with permission from Cassin B, ed. *Fundamentals for Ophthalmic Technical Personnel.* Philadelphia, PA: WB Saunders; 1995.)

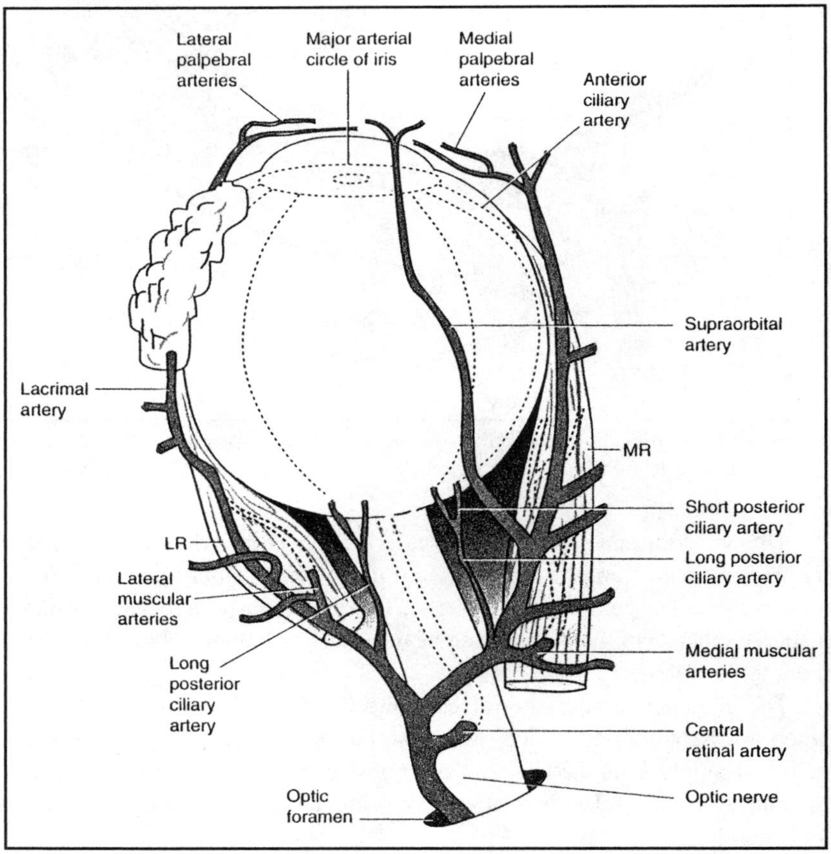

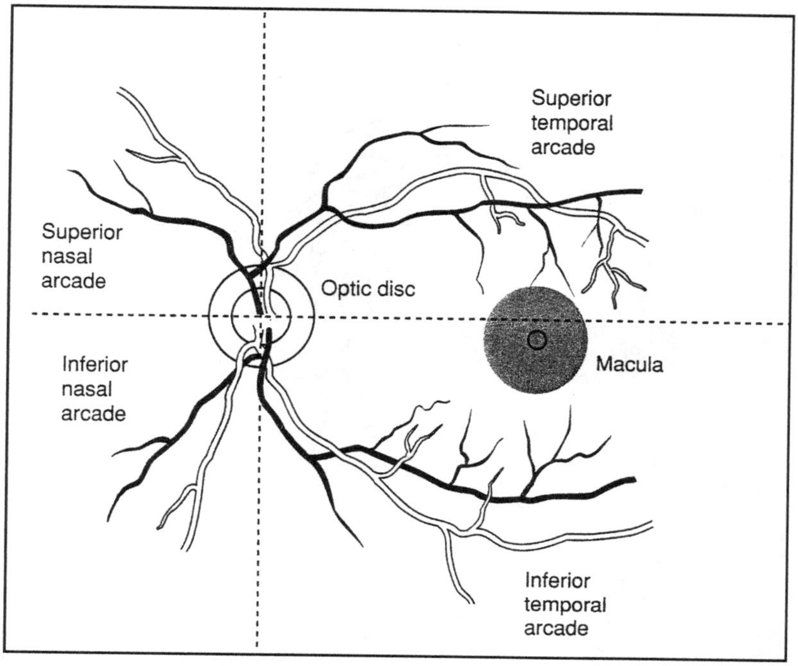

Figure 12-4. CRA and its branches. (Reprinted with permission from Cassin B, ed. *Fundamentals for Ophthalmic Technical Personnel.* Philadelphia, PA: WB Saunders; 1995.)

Venous Drainage from the Eye

Radial episcleral collecting veins receive blood from the anterior conjunctiva, limbal arcades, anterior episcleral veins, and perforating scleral veins. The episcleral collecting veins then form the anterior ciliary veins, which leave the globe anteriorly over the rectus muscles. Posteriorly, four to seven vortex veins drain the venous system (the choroid, ciliary body, and iris) into the superior and inferior ophthalmic veins (see Figure 12-1).

The diameter of the CRV is approximately 33% larger than the CRA. The superior and inferior branch veins join to form the CRV near the lamina cribrosa. The CRV pierces the dura posterior to the artery and drains into the superior ophthalmic vein and/or the cavernous sinus.

Blood from the ophthalmic veins is taken to the internal jugular vein that descends alongside the internal carotid artery. The junction of the internal jugular vein and the subclavian vein forms the brachiocephalic vein. The union of the two brachiocephalic veins forms the superior vena cava that delivers blood to the heart.

Lymphatic System

Lymph is an alkaline fluid found in tissue spaces all over the body. The lymphatic system carries lymph from the tissues to the bloodstream. The system consists of the lymph capillaries, lymph nodes, lymph vessels, and ducts. The cardiovascular system cannot function without the lymphatic system, and the immune system would be drastically impaired without it. Lymphatic capillaries capture the lymph from the tissues and deliver it back to the blood. These capillaries also transport cell debris and pathogens when tissues are inflamed.

A lymph node is a small structure enclosed in a capsule consisting of accumulations of lymphatic tissue. Lymph nodes are normally about 1 cm in diameter. They produce lymphocytes and monocytes (cells involved in fighting infection). As lymph passes through the nodes, particulate matter (such as bacteria) is filtered out to prevent it from entering the bloodstream. Nodes can

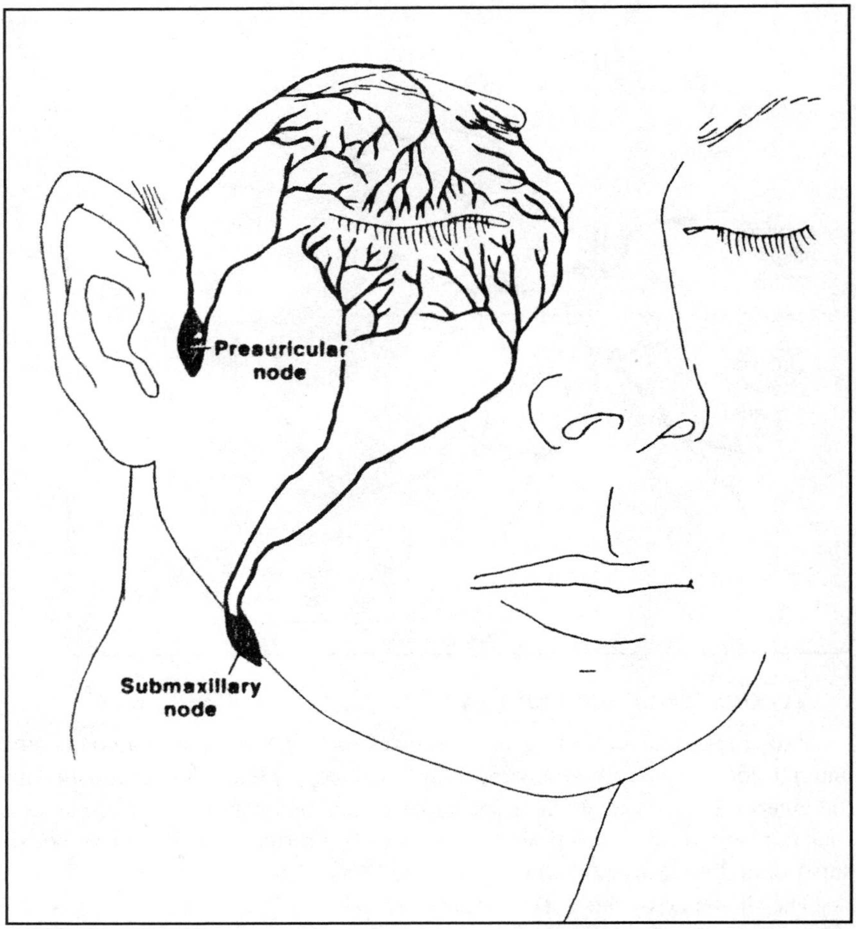

Figure 12-5. Lymphatic system of the eyelids. (Reprinted with permission from Meltzer MA. *Ophthalmic Plastic Surgery for the General Ophthalmologist.* Baltimore, MD: Williams and Wilkins; 1979.)

occur singly or in groups. The most notable groups are in the neck (cervical lymph nodes), armpit (axillary lymph nodes), and the groin (inguinal lymph nodes).

The preauricular node, located in front of the ear, is the first interceptor station of the lymphatic drainage system from the lids and conjunctiva (Figure 12-5). When the preauricular node becomes tender or palpable, it can be used as an index of the severity of the infectious process (usually viral) involving the lids or conjunctiva.

Similar to the venous system, the lymphatic capillaries join larger, thicker-walled vessels. Eventually, all lymph is delivered into the venous system at the junction of the subclavian and internal jugular veins.

Immune System

The immune system, including the lymphatic and cardiovascular organs, protects the body from foreign substances (antigens). The health of the body relies on the immune system, which consists of nonspecific and specific body defenses for recognizing and repelling antigens. Nonspecific defenses are effective against all foreign substances. Specific defenses must be exposed to the antigen before developing a defense against it.

Part of the nonspecific defenses are surface membrane barriers, specifically the skin, tears, mucus, and saliva. A cornea with an intact epithelium is rarely prone to infection. The risk of infection increases when the epithelium is compromised or the tear film is deficient. The tear film contains antibacterial and antiviral proteins that contribute to the nonspecific defense. Another part of the nonspecific defense is the rapid inflammation of tissue that takes place after injury or infection.

Specific, or adaptive, immunity is the body's defense against antigens that were able to penetrate the nonspecific defenses. This defense system tailors its response to act only on a specific type of invader. It also has a "memory" to provide a better response upon repeat exposure to the same antigen. The adaptive immune response consists of two types: humoral and cell-mediated.

Humoral immunity is provided by antibodies produced by lymphocytes (B cells). These cells circulate in the body's fluids (humors) and bind to pathogens. Then, with the aid of helper T cells, the lymphocytes transform into blast cells. Blast cells divide rapidly to form a clone of identical cells. Some of the blast cells serve as memory cells for future invasions by the same antigen. Others transform into antibody-producing plasma cells. The antibodies (immunoglobulins) then bind to the antigen. Some antibodies neutralize the antigen, while others mark the antigen for a chemical reaction with the complement system (a group of blood proteins). Complement will then either cause the antigen to burst or attract phagocytes to destroy it.

Cell-mediated immunity involves production of non-antibody–producing lymphocytes by the thymus (T cells). Helper T cells release chemical mediators to aid the inflammatory response or to activate lymphocytes or macrophages. Killer T cells attack and destroy body cells infected by intracellular parasites.

It is possible that the immune system will malfunction, decreasing its effectiveness or damaging the body. A depressed immune system is known as immunodeficient. Damage to the body by the immune system can be caused by allergies (hypersensitivity), immunological tolerances (failure to respond to a previously encountered antigen), and autoimmune disease (producing antibodies against the body's own tissue).

The immune system is responsible for the rejection of transplanted tissue when it mistakes the graft for a harmful intruder. This is more likely to occur when the graft contains blood. However, even the avascular cornea is subject to rejection by the host. Ninety percent of corneal transplants are successful; 10% are rejected. Steroid drops are often used to compromise the immune system after the signs of rejection (redness, photophobia, decreased vision, and pain) occur. This manages to salvage the transplant in most cases.

Infants and children have had limited exposure to antigens, and therefore have a less powerful immune system than a typical adult. Eye infections, such as conjunctivitis, are quite common among children and can be easily transmitted to other children in environments such as a daycare facility. Conversely, the immune system tends to lose its effectiveness with age. This factor puts elderly individuals at greater risk of immunodeficiency and autoimmune diseases and allows for the spread of disease within nursing homes.

Vaccines are used to prepare the immune system to fight certain diseases. The body is injected with a weaker form of the disease, so that the body can identify it and form antibodies. Then, if the antigens responsible for the disease penetrate the body at a later date, the body has sufficient antibodies to combat the foreign invaders. Haemophilus influenza B (HiB) vaccine is used to decrease the childhood risk of orbital cellulitis caused by Haemophilus disease. Vaccines have also been effective against diseases such as tetanus, diphtheria, and polio. Due to the nature of vaccines, they are not useful once the disease has already been contracted.

Glossary of Common Disorders

branch retinal vein occlusion (BRVO): Partial or complete blockage in one of the branches of the retinal vein causing varying degrees of visual loss, most common in elderly or those with hypertensive retinopathy. Hemorrhages and retinal edema occur in the affected area.

branch retinal artery occlusion (BRAO): Partial or complete blockage in one of the branches of the retinal artery. The retina in the affected area appears white. The patient may or may not notice visual loss depending on how much of the retina is affected.

central retinal vein occlusion (CRVO): Partial or complete blockage of the central retinal vein. In milder (nonischemic) cases, there is good prognosis for recovery. Ischemic cases will have extensive retinal hemorrhages, visual loss, afferent pupillary defect, and may develop secondary glaucoma.

central retinal artery occlusion (CRAO): Partial or complete blockage of the central retinal artery. Patient will report painless loss of vision and will present with afferent pupillary defect. A "cherry red spot" is seen at the fovea, which is still supplied with blood via the ciliary artery. Immediate treatment is required, but even then, prognosis is poor for visual recovery.

retinopathy, diabetic: Damage to the retina due to circulatory problems in the retinal vasculature caused by diabetes. More likely to occur in poorly controlled disease. The earliest phase is background diabetic retinopathy. In this phase, the arteries in the retina become weakened and leak, forming small, dot-like hemorrhages. These leaking vessels often lead to swelling or edema in the retina and decreased vision. Proliferative diabetic retinopathy occurs when oxygen-deprived parts of the retina develop new blood vessels that tend to leak easily.

retinopathy, hypertensive: Caused by high blood pressure. Whereas diabetic retinopathy presents with a “wet” retina (multiple hemorrhages, multiple exudates, and extensive edema), hypertensive retinopathy has a “dry” retina (few hemorrhages, rare edema, rare exudate, but multiple cotton-wool spots). Advanced cases may develop a macular star (ring of exudates from the macula to the disc).

Chapter 13

Inflammatory Response

Al Lens, COMT

KEY POINTS

- Inflammation is a response to infection or injury. It occurs as a normal part of the immune response.
- The components of inflammation are redness, heat, swelling, and pain.
- Infection and inflammation can occur individually.
- Infected or injured cells release chemicals, most notably histamines and prostaglandins, to promote inflammation.
- Complement is a very effective chemical defense mechanism consisting of more than a dozen different blood-borne proteins.
- Fever is part of the body's defense system. The increased temperature inhibits microbial growth.

Definition and Purpose

Inflammation is a nonspecific immune response that occurs as a reaction to any type of bodily injury. Its purpose is to destroy the invading organism or control damage so that tissue repair can begin. While inflammation can occur as a result of infection, the two terms should not be confused; it is possible for one to occur without the other.

Despite its healing qualities, inflammation can also be harmful. Scar formation can occur, or the body can become hypersensitive to certain antigens. Inflammation can also become chronic, such as rheumatoid arthritis in the body or recurrent iritis in the eye.

The typical signs of inflammation include redness, swelling, heat, and pain. Extensive inflammation may be accompanied by fever. Redness and heat are local reactions caused by dilation of the blood vessels, which increases blood flow. The vessels then become more permeable and allow plasma to escape from the capillaries into the tissues, causing edema (swelling). The excessive fluid pressing on nerve endings causes pain.

Diseases with "itis" as their suffix involve inflammation (ie, the name of the disease usually identifies the inflamed tissue). For example, conjunctivitis is inflammation of the conjunctiva, iritis is inflammation of the iris, and keratitis refers to inflammation of the cornea.

Inflammatory Process

Inflammation is a complex response involving numerous components (Figure 13-1). It is closely linked to the immune system, which was discussed in the last chapter. The process is essentially the same whether the affected part is the eye or some other structure. During the inflammatory process, various blood cells move into the injured tissues (Figure 13-2 and Table 13-1). Chemical mediators, such as complement, histamine, metabolites, prostaglandins, and kinins, are released by white blood cells and tissues to continue the inflammatory response. Modifications are made to the response according to what produced the inflammation.

Complement

Complement is a group of more than a dozen proteins in the blood. Although part of the B cell-mediated immune response, complement also influences the inflammatory process. Some of the proteins in complement stimulate the release of histamine. Others increase the white blood cell count in the area, enhancing phagocytosis (the cell's ingestion and digestion of bacteria and particles). Yet another function of complement is to coat the antigen with a substance that makes it easier for macrophages (cells capable of phagocytosis) to stick to the invader.

Histamine

Histamine is a chemical that plays an important role in the inflammatory process. The release of histamine increases gastric secretion, contracts bronchial smooth muscle, and dilates capillaries. In the body, histamine is synthesized in mast cells where it stays resident, along with serotonin, until it is released in response to chemical or physical injury. Dilation of the blood vessels is accompanied by decreased blood pressure and increased permeability of the vessel walls. Fluids can then escape into the surrounding tissue, causing swelling. In the eye, this can cause itchiness, tearing, conjunctival edema, and swelling of the lids. Antihistamine drugs are useful to counteract the effects of histamine.

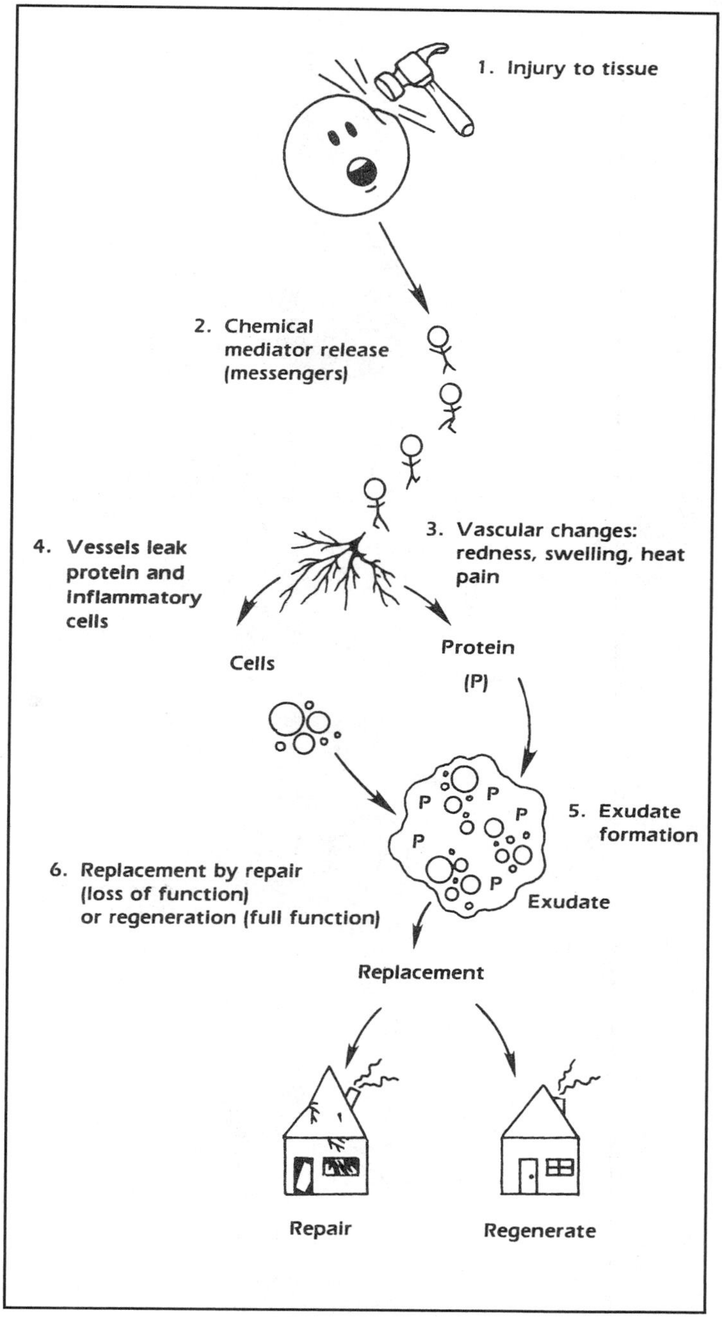
1. Injury to tissue
2. Chemical mediator release (messengers)
3. Vascular changes: redness, swelling, heat pain
4. Vessels leak protein and inflammatory cells
Cells
Protein (P)
P
5. Exudate formation
Exudate
6. Replacement by repair (loss of function) or regeneration (full function)
Replacement
Repair
Regenerate

Figure 13-1. Schematic of the inflammatory pathway. (Reprinted with permission from Nemeth SC, Shea CA. *Medical Sciences for the Ophthalmic Assistant.* Thorofare, NJ: SLACK Incorporated; 1988.)

Figure 13-2. Inflammatory cells. (Reprinted with permission from Nemeth SC, Shea CA. *Medical Sciences for the Ophthalmic Assistant.* Thorofare, NJ: SLACK Incorporated; 1988.)

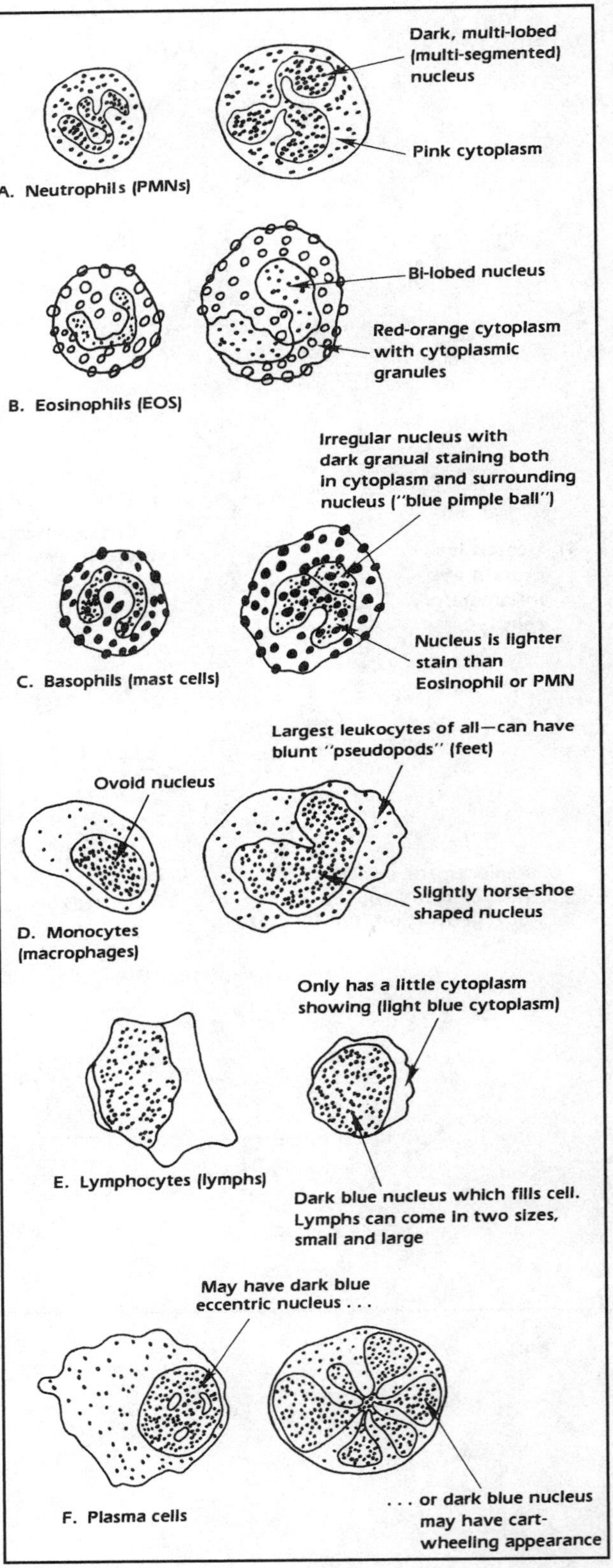

Table 13-1
Inflammatory Cells

Neutrophil (also called polymorphonucleocyte, "poly," or PMN)
Appearance: Multi-lobed nucleus with pink cytoplasm.
Function: They are the first line of defense in inflammation. They release enzymes, eat bacteria, and are seen in any case of inflammation—especially in bacterial infections.

Eosinophil (EOS)
Appearance: Bi-lobed nucleus with red-orange cytoplasm.
Function: They are the chief cell in allergic inflammation and are associated with parasites.

Basophil (mast cell)
Appearance: Dark granular-stained nucleus with blue cytoplasm, looks like blue pimple ball.
Function: Basophils contain histamine, which causes vasodilation leading to chemosis and edema. It causes the hypersensitivity reaction seen in giant papillary conjunctivitis (GPC), allergy, and atopic dermatitis.

Lymphocyte (lymph)
Appearance: They look like small blue balls with dark blue nuclei. Only a little cytoplasm shows.
Function: They are the chief cell in chronic inflammation.

Plasma cell
Appearance: Eccentric nucleus; looks like a large lymph with dark blue nucleus pushed to the side (the nucleus may have a cart-wheeling appearance).
Function: Plasma cells arise from B-lymphocytes. Their function is the production of antibodies.

Monocyte (macrophage or histiocyte)
Appearance: One large ovoid or horseshoe-shaped blue nucleus with dull gray-blue cytoplasm (much larger than the lymphocyte).
Function: It is the major phagocytic cell in the body.

Epithelioid cell
Appearance: Kidney-shaped nucleus with pink cytoplasm.
Function: In granulomatous disease, monocytes may be converted into epithelioid cells. They join together to form giant cells with 3 to 6 nuclei. Seen in sarcoid, trachoma, and viral infections.

Reprinted with permission from Nemeth SC, Shea CA. Medical Sciences for the Ophthalmic Assistant. *Thorofare, NJ: SLACK Incorporated; 1988.*

Metabolites

Metabolites are the product of energy and material transformations that occur within living cells (metabolism). Metabolites are involved in two fundamental processes—anabolism and catabolism. Anabolism is a constructive process that takes a nonliving substance from the blood and converts it into the living cytoplasm of a cell. Catabolism is a destructive process that takes a complex substance and converts it into simpler substances, usually with the release of energy.

Prostaglandins

Prostaglandins are unsaturated fatty acids that form quickly, exert their effects locally, and then decay or are destroyed by enzymes in the lungs. In the inflammatory process, prostaglandins can cause constriction or dilation of blood vessels and bronchodilation in the lungs, and can increase sensitivity to pain. Thromboxane is a type of prostaglandin that plays an important role in the aggregation and release of platelets and is a potent vasoconstrictor. The activation of platelets can lead to further production of thromboxane.

Kinins

Kinins are inflammatory mediators that are capable of increasing the blood flow and permeability of small blood vessels. Kinins act to increase prostaglandin production. Bradykinin, one of the kinins, is a very potent vasodilator that increases permeability of postcapillary venules. It can also influence smooth muscle contraction and incite pain.

Interleukin-1 aids the communication between the cells of the immune system. This helps to coordinate the immune response and regulates the activity of T- and B-lymphocytes. Interleukin-1 can cause fever, decrease the levels of iron in the blood, and increase the production of leukocytes. Fever contributes to the defense mechanism of the body by inhibiting the growth of microorganisms. However, a very high fever can be counterproductive because the excessive heat can inactivate critical enzymes. Decreasing the level of iron in the blood is beneficial in the case of bacterial infection because bacteria depend on large amounts of iron to grow. Leukocytes act as scavengers, helping to combat infection. In the case of a virus, leukocytes may release interferon, a chemical that inhibits the production of the virus. This prevents the virus from spreading to other cells and enhances the activity of cells that destroy the virus.

Ocular Inflammation

The eye and surrounding tissues are susceptible to inflammation. The ocular tissue that is most commonly associated with inflammation is the conjunctiva. Conjunctivitis is more common among individuals who wear soft contact lenses but can occur in anyone. Giant papillary conjunctivitis (GPC) causes papillae in the conjunctiva of the eyelids. Follicular conjunctivitis is characterized by hundreds of follicles (elevations composed of lymphoid tissue). Other sources of conjunctivitis include allergy, bacteria, and viruses.

Inflammation that spreads through the orbital tissue is called orbital cellulitis. Bacteria, usually *streptococci* or *staphylococci,* are often the cause of the inflammation. Signs of orbital cellulitis include itching or a burning sensation, decreased vision, proptosis (bulging forward of the eye), limitation of eye movement, painful swelling of the upper and lower lids (upper is usually greater), decreased eyelid and corneal sensation, and general malaise (feeling unwell).

The cornea can become involved in various forms of inflammation. Keratitis is characterized by a loss of luster and transparency as well as infiltrates (aggregates of inflammatory cells beneath the epithelium). Inflammation of the cornea can be caused by something as simple as drying. Dendritic keratitis is characteristic of viral infections. Keratic precipitates on the endothelium are inflammatory cells from the anterior chamber that adhere to the inside layer of the cornea.

Iritis causes protein and white blood cells to be released into the anterior chamber. Patients suffering from iritis will complain of pain, blurred vision, and tearing. A red eye and small pupil are also noted. Uveitis is an inflammation of any of the structures of the uveal tract (iris, ciliary body, and choroid). Severe inflammation within the eye can cause a hypopyon, an accumulation of pus in the lower aspect of the anterior chamber. Inflammation of the retina, or retinitis, can cause loss of vision, leading to blindness.

For more on ocular inflammations and infections, please refer to the Basic Bookshelf title *Overview of Ocular Disorders.*

Glossary of Common Disorders

blepharitis: *See* Glossary of Common Disorders (GCD), Chapter 4.
canaliculitis: *See* GCD, Chapter 4.
chorioretinitis: *See* GCD, Chapter 9.
conjunctivitis: *See* GCD, Chapter 6.
dacryocystitis: *See* GCD, Chapter 4.
endophthalmitis: *See* GCD, Chapters 5,9.
episcleritis: *See* GCD, Chapter 6.
iritis: *See* anterior uveitis/iritis, GCD, Chapter 8.
keratitis: *See* GCD, Chapter 7.
retinitis: *See* GCD, Chapter 9.
scleritis: *See* GCD, Chapter 6.
uveitis, anterior (iritis): *See* anterior uveitis/iritis, GCD, Chapter 8.
uveitis, posterior: *See* GCD, Chapter 9.
vitritis: *See* GCD, Chapter 9.

Chapter 14

Binocular Vision

Al Lens, COMT

KEY POINTS

- The position of the eyes in the skull allows their visual field to overlap considerably.
- Binocular depth perception, or stereopsis, uses retinal disparity to provide the most powerful binocular depth cue.
- The only real advantage of binocular vision is stereopsis.
- Stereo acuity is measured in seconds of arc.
- High level stereo acuity develops between 5 and 9 years of age.

Requirements

"Normal vision" is the presence of 20/20 visual acuity in both eyes and the ability to use the eyes together (binocular vision). Several requirements must be met in order to have normal binocular vision—the body must be equipped with two functioning eyes with visual fields that overlap considerably, both eyes must be able to maintain fixation on an object (misalignment of the eyes is not conducive to single binocular vision), both eyes must have normal (or close to normal) vision, the retinal image from both eyes must be of similar size and shape, and the brain must be able to blend the slightly dissimilar images into a single image. The only real advantage of binocular vision appears to be stereopsis (visual perception of solidity and depth).

Binocular vision is developed after birth. The human visual system learns how to blend the two images in various stages. First, there must be accurate alignment of the two eyes. Then the brain must recognize that the images are similar and learn how to blend the two images together. Next, the brain must learn to maintain the blending, even when the object is moved off the fovea. Finally, stereo acuity is developed. High level stereo acuity seems to develop between 5 and 9 years of age.

Overlapping Fields

The position of the eyes in the skull allows their visual field to overlap considerably. Stereopsis is only possible if there is overlap in the visual fields. It is the slightly dissimilar image from each eye that provides stereopsis; if there is no overlap, then the image from each eye would be entirely different, preventing the brain from blending the two images together.

The visual field of each eye, in primary gaze, extends approximately 60 degrees nasally from fixation and about 90 degrees temporally. This provides a binocular field (the field of vision of both eyes that overlap) of 120 degrees (Figure 14-1). Due to the anatomical features of the face, the binocular field will vary somewhat depending on the position of gaze (ie, the nose limits the nasal field of vision).

As discussed in Chapter 9, the nerve fibers representing the left side of each retina remain on the left side of the visual pathway. The semidecussation that occurs in the optic chiasm allows the nerve fibers representing corresponding retinal points to join each other in the visual pathway. This is an important feature in our ability to perceive depth. Corresponding retinal points, or the points on both retinas that have the same visual direction, send their nerve impulses to the same point in the visual cortex and provide fusion (see below).

Fusion

Fusion is the blending of two similar images (one from each retina) into a single image that is maintained as the eyes converge or diverge. Central fusion relates to the image from the macula of each eye. Peripheral fusion is the blending of similar images from the peripheral areas of both eyes.

Fusion can be separated into three grades—first grade fusion is the basic ability to superimpose the two dissimilar images and perceive them as one image, second grade fusion (fusion with amplitude) is the ability of the brain to maintain blending of the dissimilar images as the images move off the fovea, and third grade fusion is the perception of depth.

An imaginary arc in space, called a horopter, contains points whose images fall on corresponding retinal points (when a central point is imaged on both fovea) (Figure 14-2). Any object

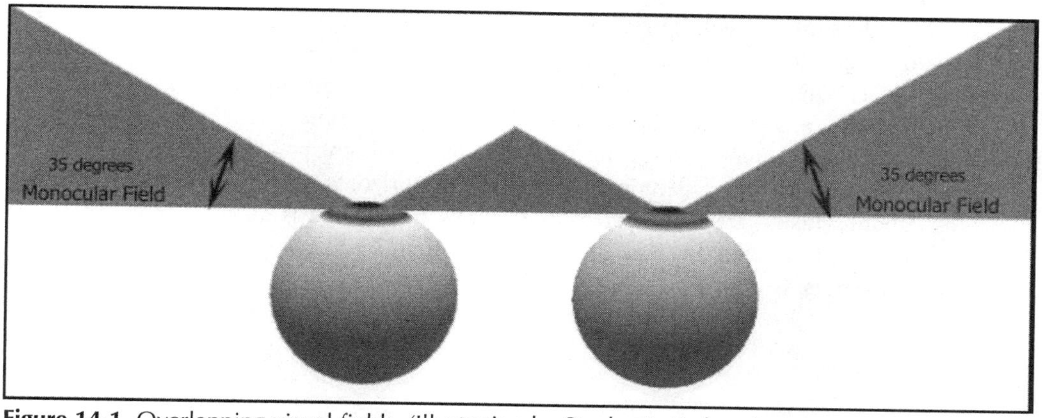

Figure 14-1. Overlapping visual fields. (Illustration by Stephanie Embrey.)

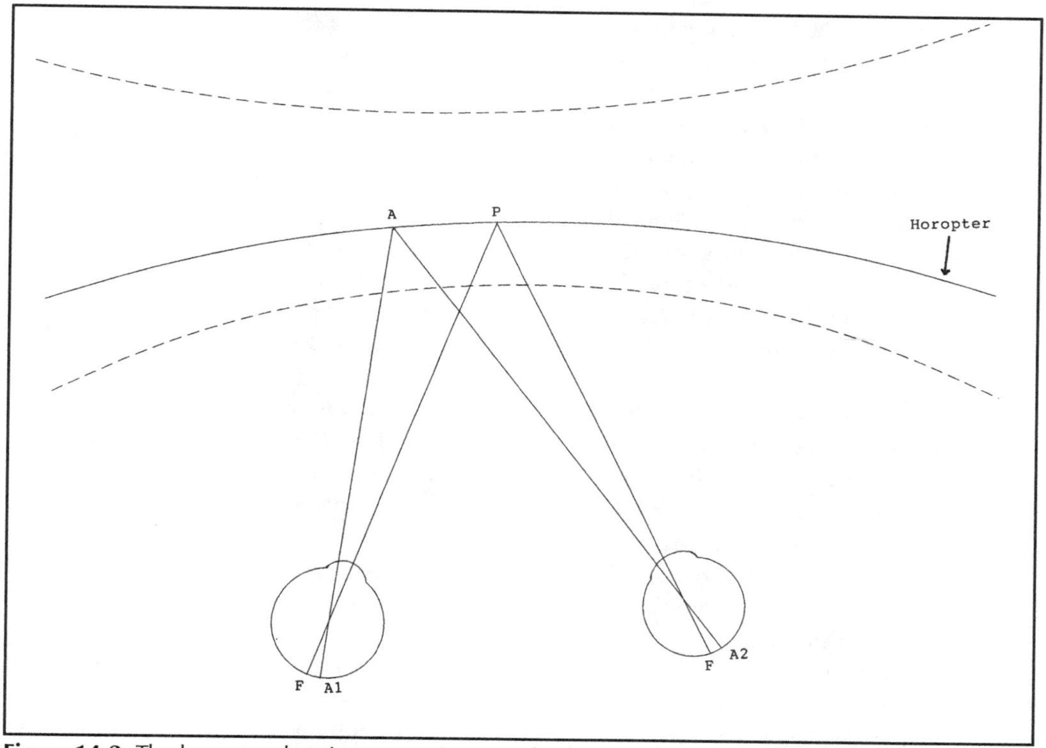

Figure 14-2. The horopter showing two points (P—the fixation point, and A) and their corresponding retinal points in each eye (F—the fovea, A1 and A2). Panum's fusional space lies between the dotted lines. (Drawing courtesy of Jan Ledford, COMT.)

that lies along the horopter will be seen singly. The image of objects in front of or behind the horopter will be seen double since the image will not be on corresponding retinal points. Diplopia caused by objects lying outside the horopter is known as physiologic diplopia.

An important point to consider is that a small area exists in front of and behind the horopter that defies physiologic diplopia, allowing fusion despite noncorresponding retinal points. This is the phenomenon that allows stereopsis to occur. The horizontal area outside the horopter is known as Panum's fusion area. The extent of Panum's fusion area is about 15 minutes of arc (7 minutes of arc in front of and behind the point of fixation). The size of Panum's area increases with distance from the fovea.

Stereopsis

Binocular depth perception, or stereopsis, uses retinal disparity to provide the most powerful binocular depth cue. While monocular vision can provide many cues regarding depth perception, it does not provide the full experience of depth—as does stereopsis (binocular depth perception). The human brain synthesizes information about depth and distance from numerous sources. Monocular cues include relative size of the image, superposition, convergence of lines, accommodation, and motion parallax. Binocular cues include retinal disparity and convergence of the eyes.

If a person is familiar with an object, its size can provide clues regarding its distance. Logically, the smaller the image, the further away the object must be. Superposition is the overlapping of two or more objects; an object that obscures another is perceived as being closer. Lines, such as those representing the edges of a road, converge with increasing distance. Impulses sent from the ciliary muscle provide information about the amount of accommodation being used; the more accommodation being expended, the closer the object must be. The brain compares speeds of moving objects to judge their distance; objects that are nearby pass the viewer more rapidly than distant objects.

Stereopsis produces a three-dimensional view of objects. Because it relies on retinal disparity, stereopsis is only effective when viewing objects within 20 feet. Beyond this distance, there is negligible difference between the image seen by the two eyes, and stereopsis is almost nonexistent. The retinal disparity must be horizontal since vertical disparities do not yield stereopsis. (The eyes are beside each other, not arranged vertically.)

Stereo acuity is measured in seconds of arc. There are 360 degrees in a circle, each degree separated into 60 minutes. Each minute is further divided into 60 seconds. Therefore, there are 360 seconds of arc in a single degree.

Normal central stereopsis, or stereo acuity at the fovea, is 67 seconds of arc or less. Stereopsis diminishes quickly as the stimulus is moved into the periphery. Stereo acuity is considered quite poor beyond 20 degrees of fixation. (Tests to measure stereo acuity in the clinic are described in the Basic Bookshelf title *Clinical Skills for the Ophthalmic Examination: Basic Procedures.*)

Stereo acuity, like visual acuity, must be developed during childhood. It cannot be learned later in life. Therefore, vision and ocular alignment must be normal as a child. Occlusion therapy, used to treat amblyopia, can adversely affect stereopsis. However, it is more important to improve the child's vision, as decreased visual acuity will also prevent normal stereopsis.

Chapter 15

Physiologic Optics

Al Lens, COMT

KEY POINTS

- The speed of light in air is almost the same as the speed of light in a vacuum.
- Light striking a medium perpendicular to its surface will not be bent, regardless of the index of refraction.
- The overall refractive index of the eye is 1.33.
- The overall power of the eye is 58.64 diopters.
- The amplitude of accommodation decreases with age, leading to a condition called presbyopia.

Index of Refraction

The speed with which light passes through a medium is represented by the refractive index (or index of refraction). The higher the refractive index of a given material, the slower light is able to pass through. The refractive index can be determined by dividing the speed of light in the new substance into the speed of light in a vacuum. (The speed of light in air is almost the same as that in a vacuum, but there is a slight difference. Therefore, to be technically correct, one should refer to the refractive index that is obtained using the speed of light in air as the *relative refractive index*.) For example, if the speed of light in the medium is 140,000 miles/second, and the speed of light in a vacuum is 186,000 miles/second, then the refractive index of the medium is 1.33 (186,000 divided by 140,000).

The refractive index of a medium determines how light will be bent when it enters the medium at an angle. (Light striking the medium perpendicular to the surface will not be bent, regardless of the index of refraction.) Material with a high refractive index will bend light more than a medium with a lower refractive index. Therefore, when light travels through a vacuum (refractive index of 1.00) and enters a lens (refractive index greater than 1.00), light will be bent toward the surface (Figure 15-1).

The refractive power of a structure is determined by its shape and the refractive index of the medium itself, as well as that of the surrounding media. For example, a round piece of solid glass has considerable refractive power. An hollow glass cylinder has insignificant refractive power, but once it is filled with water, it provides shape for the water. Now the cylinder has a refractive power similar to the solid glass tube. Furthermore, a lens will lose its power when it is immersed in a fluid that has the same refractive index.

Refractive Power of Media

The overall refractive index of the eye is 1.33. However, the eye consists of an optical system with various indices of refraction—the cornea's refractive index is 1.376; aqueous, tears, and vitreous have a refractive index of 1.3337; and the noncataractous lens has a refractive index of 1.41 in the nucleus and 1.38 in the cortex.

The radius of the curvature for the average cornea is 7.8 mm on the anterior surface. This convex (plus) curvature, combined with a refractive index of 1.376, gives the central anterior cornea a refractive power of 48.8 diopters. The posterior surface of the cornea is concave (minus) in shape, reducing the overall power of the cornea by 5.8 diopters. Thus, the overall power of the average cornea is 43.0 diopters. It is important to note that if the cornea is removed from the eye, it has little refractive power because the anterior and posterior curves are quite similar. The power of the cornea is, in large part, due to the shape it provides for the aqueous.

The refractive power of the crystalline lens tends to change with age as its shape and refractive index changes. The average power of the lens is 15 diopters. The power can also be changed (temporarily) by accommodation.

The vitreous body magnifies the image to be formed on the retina, contributing significantly to the refractive status of the eye. If the vitreous is surgically removed, it must be replaced by a substance with similar refractive index to maintain the overall focusing power of the eye.

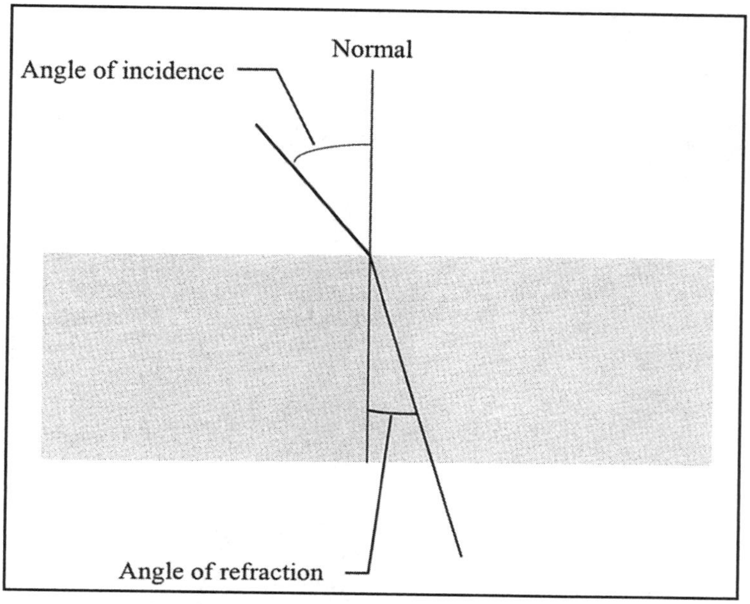

Figure 15-1. Index of refraction.

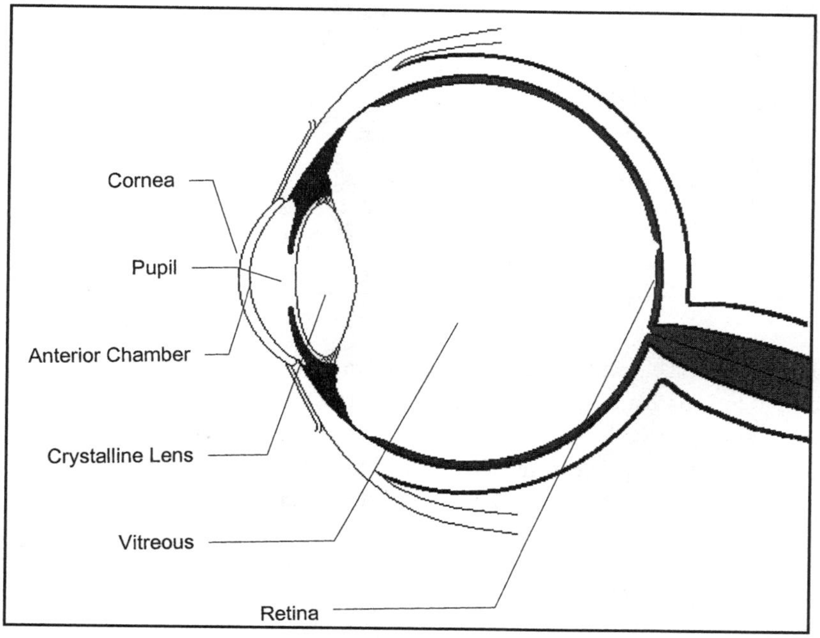

Figure 15-2. Pathway of light through the human eye.

Pathway of Light

As light enters the eye, it first passes through the tear film. It then enters the cornea, followed by the anterior chamber (AC) filled with aqueous humor. The iris separates the AC and posterior chambers and light enters the posterior chamber through the pupil. From here, light travels through the crystalline lens, then the vitreous cavity. Finally, light stimulates the photoreceptors which lie within the retina (Figure 15-2). Because of the refractive power of the eye, the image is inverted on the retina. The optic nerve carries the impulses from the retina to the brain, where the image is finally seen.

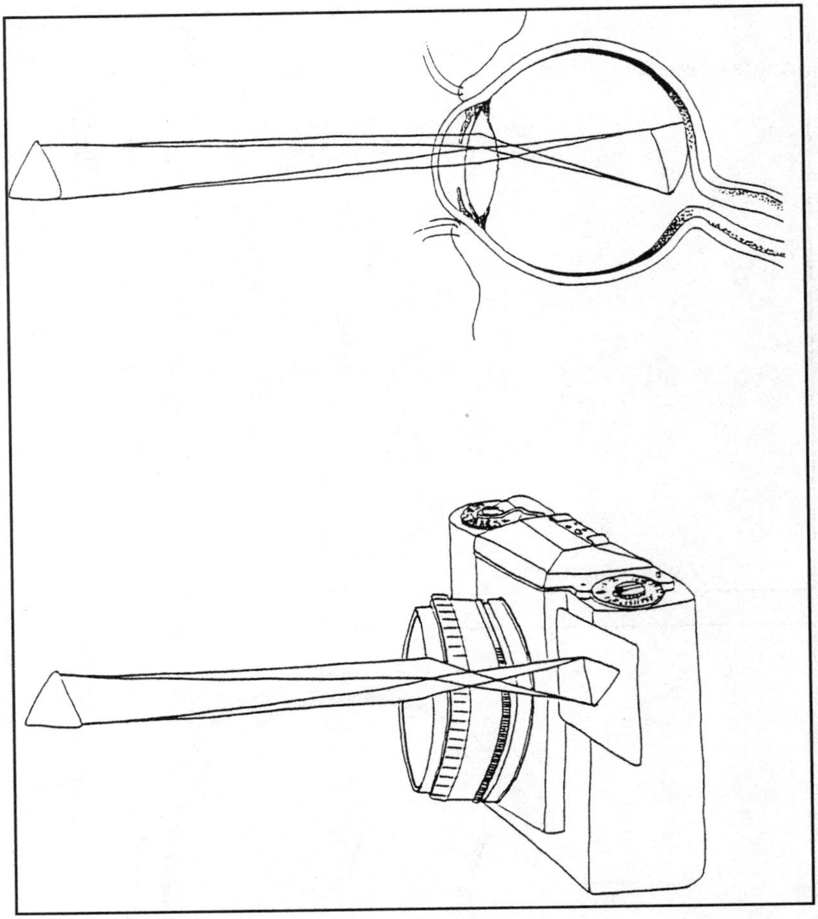

Figure 15-3. The eye compared to a camera. (Drawing by Holly Hess Smith. Reprinted with permission from Gayton JL, Ledford JK. *The Crystal Clear Guide to Sight for Life*. Lancaster, Pa: Starburst Publishers; 1996.)

In many ways, the eye is like a camera (Figure 15-3). The lenses of the camera are similar to the optic media (fluids and transparent tissues) of the eye. Film in a camera is comparable to the retina of the eye where the image is collected. Film is sent away to a lab for processing, and the retina sends its image to the brain for processing. The lab will print the pictures upright, and the brain will form an upright image from the inverted image on the retina.

Schematic Eye

The schematic eye of Gullstrand (Figure 15-4) is a model that uses average values for the optical system of the eye. The primary focal length is 15.70 mm and the secondary focal length (corneal apex to retina) is 24.38 mm. The primary and secondary principle planes are located 1.35 mm and 1.60 mm from the corneal apex, respectively. The primary principle plane is the position that rays of light entering the eye could be considered as refracted by a single, thin lens. The same applies to the secondary principle plane, except it relates to rays of light leaving the eye. The nodal points are located 7.08 mm and 7.33 mm from the corneal apex. Nodal points are a pair of points located on the axis of the eye's optical system such that a ray of light entering the eye directed toward the primary nodal point leaves the eye as though it passed through the secondary nodal point. The

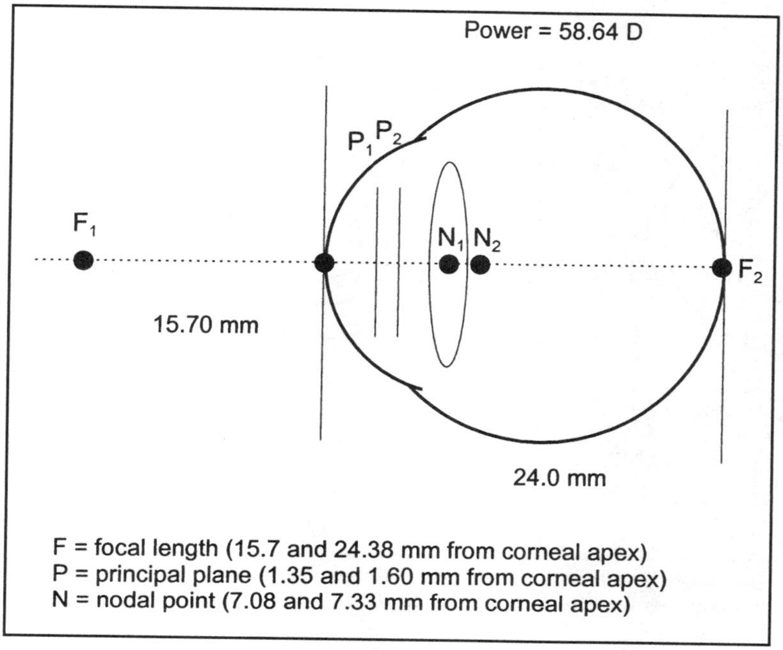

Figure 15-4. Schematic eye of Gullstrand.

power of the eye's optical system is 58.64 diopters, with the majority of the power coming from the cornea (43.05 diopters) and the lens (19.11 diopters).

The schematic eye is used as a general reference for determining mathematical values. However, it makes certain assumptions that can lead to inaccuracies if the values in the schematic eye are accepted as true. For further information on this topic, see Basic Bookshelf title *Optics, Retinoscopy, and Refractometry, Second Edition*.

Accommodative Process

The crystalline lens of the eye is capable of changing its shape with the help of the ciliary muscle. About 70 thread-like fibers, known as zonules, extend from the ciliary muscle to the lens capsule. As the ciliary muscle contracts, it relaxes the tension on the zonules (Figure 15-5). This results in increased curvature and power of the crystalline lens (accommodation). Most of the change in curvature is due to the anterior surface of the lens moving forward. Other changes occur in the lens during accommodation, including a slight change in the shape of the posterior lens surface and a gravitational tendency to sink within the globe.

The accommodative process is stimulated by either the blurred image of a nearby object or an awareness of the object's proximity. Along with a change in shape of the crystalline lens, accommodation also causes the eyes to converge and the pupils to constrict. This chain of events is known as the accommodative triad or the near response.

The relationship between the amount of accommodation and convergence is called the accommodation-convergence/accommodation (AC/A) ratio. This is an important factor in providing a clear, single image of near objects. If the amount of convergence is not appropriate for the amount of accommodation, a blurred or double image would be seen.

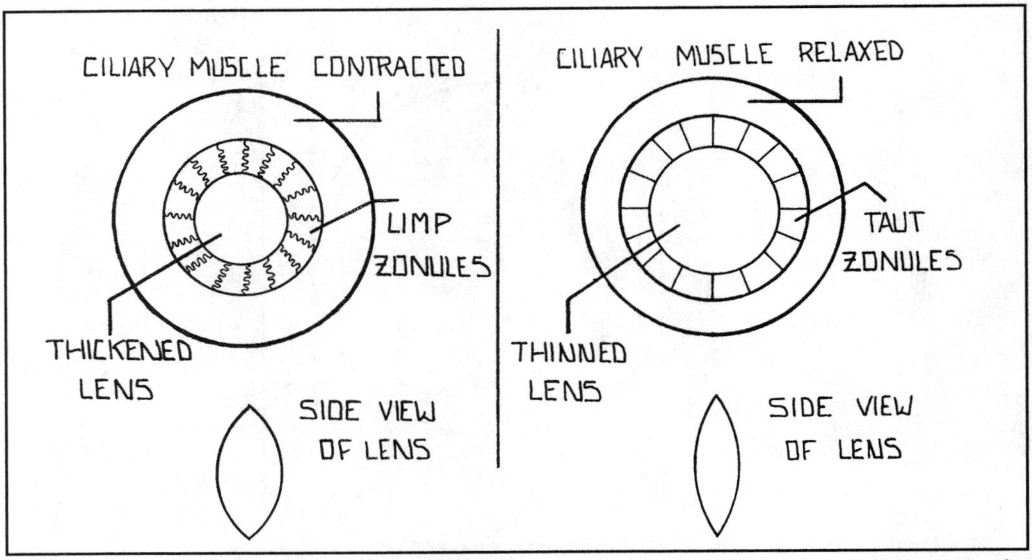

Figure 15-5. The lens and ciliary muscle in (a) accommodation and (b) relaxation. (Drawing by Holly Hess Smith. Reprinted with permission from Ledford JK. *Exercises in Refractometry.* Thorofare, NJ: SLACK Incorporated; 1990.)

The amplitude of accommodation decreases with age, leading to a condition called presbyopia—the inability to alter the eye's focus adequately enough to read at a comfortable distance. Presbyopia is discussed in Chapter 16.

Pupil Size

The normal pupil diameter ranges from 2 mm to 9 mm. Similar to the aperture of a camera lens, an opening of a smaller diameter will increase the depth of focus (the range that is in focus without altering the amount of accommodation). A pupil diameter smaller than 2 mm causes light to be bent around the edges of the pupil (diffraction). This can decrease the quality of vision due to the scattering of light. Conversely, when the pupil dilates beyond 6 mm, the image becomes distorted as the bending of light rays increases toward the edge of the lens (spherical aberration).

Light that enters the eye through the center of the pupil stimulates the retinal cones more than light that strikes them obliquely. Therefore, light entering the eye through the periphery of the pupil has less effect on vision than light passing through the pupillary center. This concept is known as the Stiles-Crawford effect (Figure 15-6).

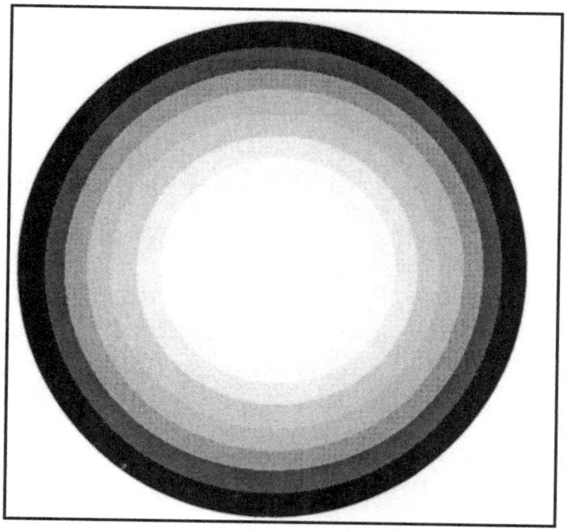

Figure 15-6. Stiles-Crawford effect: rings represent the effect of light from that area on the vision.

Chapter 16

Refractive Errors and Conditions

Al Lens, COMT

KEY POINTS

- The degree of myopia in an adult is typically reflected by the age when the first pair of corrective lenses were required—the later in life that glasses are required, the less the amount of expected myopia.
- Almost all humans are born with some degree of hyperopia.
- Astigmatism is a refractive error that is not equal in all the meridians.
- Presbyopia is a natural aging process that causes a decrease in the eye's ability to change its focus (accommodate).

Emmetropia

Emmetropia is the lack of a refractive error—the state of a "normal" eye. Light from a distant object (20 feet or more away) has essentially parallel light rays. When these light rays enter a relaxed emmetropic eye, they are focused on the retina. No lenses are required to focus the light properly. If sufficient accommodation is available, near objects will also be in focus.

There are a few conditions that must be met in order for emmetropia to exist. The power of the cornea and lens must be equal in all meridians, and the sum of their powers must be appropriate for the length (size) of the eye. The power of each refractive structure of the eye is determined by its refractive index and curvature. The refractive index of the aqueous and vitreous humors also affect how light is focused in the eye. Failure of these parameters to be synchronized will result in a refractive error, or ametropia.

Myopia

Myopia, or nearsightedness, is caused by the power of the refractive structures being too strong for the length of the eye—light comes to a focus in front of the retina (Figure 16-1). This can be related to an eye of normal length, if the eye's power is too strong. However, more commonly the eye is too long for its power. Myopia is corrected with minus-powered spherical lenses.

Generally speaking, for every millimeter that the eye is too long, 3 diopters of myopia will exist. If we assume the average eye is 24 mm, an eye that is 26 mm long (and of normal refractive power) will have approximately 6 diopters of myopia. An error in the power of the eye will essentially create a diopter-for-diopter refractive error (ie, a cornea that is 2 diopters too strong will cause 2 diopters of myopia [assuming all other parameters are normal]).

As the name nearsightedness implies, the eye is capable of seeing close objects, but distant objects will be blurry. An uncorrected myope will be able to see to read; how close the material must be held for clarity is determined by the amount of myopia. A mild myope will often prefer to read without his or her glasses. However, a person with greater than 4 diopters of myopia will usually report that the material must be held uncomfortably close and will choose to wear corrective lenses for almost all activities.

One can estimate the amount of myopia present in an eye by determining the farpoint. This is done by asking the person to indicate when fine print first becomes blurry as it is moved away from the eye. This distance (the farpoint) is measured in meters, or fractions thereof. Using the reciprocal (dividing into one), the amount of myopia in diopters is determined. For example, if the farpoint is 25 cm (0.25 meters), the amount of myopia is 4 diopters (1 divided by 0.25).

Conversely, if the amount of myopia is determined, the patient's uncorrected farpoint can be quickly calculated by taking the reciprocal of the diopter power. For example, the far point of an eye with 10 diopters of myopia will be 10 cm, or 0.1 meter (1 divided by 10).

Since the presence of myopia is related to the length of the eye, it is not surprising to note changes in the refractive error as growth is seen elsewhere in the body. Many myopes get their first pair of glasses during puberty. Typically, the degree of myopia as an adult is reflected in the age that the first pair of corrective lenses were required. A person who first requires myopic correction at age 8 would be expected to be more nearsighted as an adult than a person who did not need glasses until age 16. There are, of course, exceptions to this.

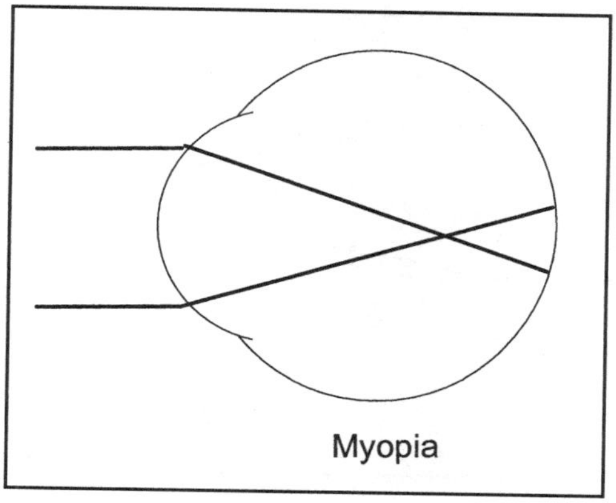

Figure 16-1. Myopia.

Some people become more myopic in dimly lit environments. This is known as night myopia and is believed to be caused by either inappropriate accommodation or spherical aberration. Low illumination limits the visibility of objects and interferes with the feedback mechanism of accommodation. Therefore, some accommodative effort is exerted despite the desire to view a distant object. Spherical aberration is caused by a large diameter pupil. (According to physics, light is bent more toward the periphery of a lens or in the case of the eye, the cornea and/or crystalline lens.) This produces positive spherical aberration, which makes the person slightly more nearsighted. When the pupil diameter is small, peripheral light does not pass through the pupil and spherical aberration is eliminated.

It is not usually possible for a person to "grow out of" myopia. Once a person is myopic, there is little hope for the refractive error to lessen as the patient ages. Also, there is not much that can be done to prevent the progression of myopia. Some people believe that advancement of myopia can be slowed by wearing contact lenses. Scientific studies do not support this theory. Orthokeratology, the practice of purposefully flattening the cornea with tight-fitting contact lenses, has been used in adults to *temporarily* reduce the amount of myopia and/or astigmatism, but it is limited to mild amounts of myopia and requires the use of a retainer lens for sustained results.

Hyperopia (Hypermetropia)

Most humans are born with some degree of hyperopia, or farsightedness. In normal eyes, emmetropia usually occurs by the age of six. However, some eyes remain too short for the focusing power of the eye (in its relaxed state), causing hyperopia. In this case, light fails to come to a focus point before reaching the retina and is focused "behind" the retina (Figure 16-2). When the eye is young, it is capable of overcoming a small to moderate amount of hyperopia using accommodation. Therefore, hyperopia may not manifest itself until later in life. Hyperopia is corrected with plus-powered spherical lenses.

Because accommodation plays an important role in how well a farsighted person can see without corrective lenses, several types of hyperopia have been identified. The amount of hyperopia that cannot be overcome by accommodation is called *absolute hyperopia*. *Manifest (or facultative) hyperopia* is the amount of hyperopia indicated by the strongest convex (plus-powered) lens accepted while retaining best visual acuity. If cycloplegic drops are used to arrest accommodation, *latent hyperopia* may be revealed (indicated by the additional convex lens accepted above the manifest result). *Total hyperopia* is the sum of the manifest and latent hyperopia.

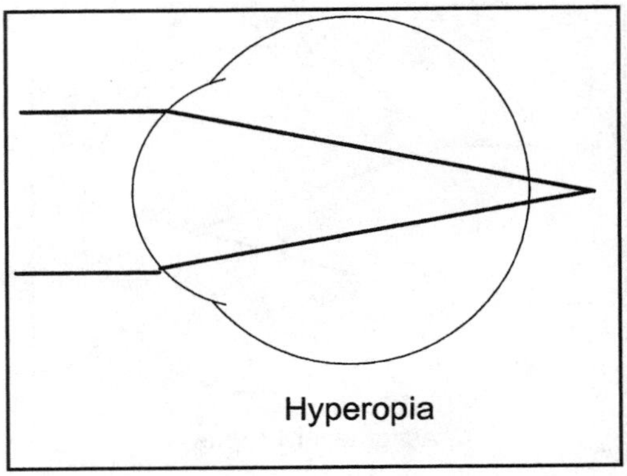

Figure 16-2. Hyperopia.

To demonstrate, consider the following example: A patient who sees 20/40 without corrective lenses and is first able to see 20/20 with a +1.00 lens has 1.00 diopter of absolute hyperopia. The same patient may accept up to +3.00 while retaining 20/20 vision; this indicates 3.00 diopters of manifest hyperopia. After the accommodation is paralyzed using cycloplegic eye drops, the patient accepts another +1.50, indicating the presence of 1.50 diopters of latent hyperopia. Total hyperopia in this example is 4.50 diopters (3.00 + 1.50).

An uncorrected hyperope will usually require reading glasses at an earlier age than an emmetrope. Later in life, when accommodation is reduced further, glasses will be required for distance as well. This is often difficult to explain to a patient since the layman's term, *farsightedness*, leads one to believe that distance vision should be good. It may be better to explain hyperopia as having *better* distance vision than near vision, and eventually glasses will be required to see clearly at all distances.

Astigmatism

Astigmatism is considered by many to be the most bothersome and confusing of the refractive errors. It is a refractive error that is not equal in all the meridians, thus the image is not focused as a single point.

In regular astigmatism, the meridians with the greatest and least amount of curvature (or refractive error) are perpendicular to each other. Instead of light being focused to a point, two focus lines are created perpendicular to each other (one focus line for each primary meridian). This causes the image to be stretched out. Regular astigmatism is corrected with a cylindrical lens. Irregular astigmatism is not entirely correctable because the refractive error changes across the pupillary aperture. This is most common in eyes with corneal pathology.

An unequally curved cornea is the usual cause of astigmatism, but it may occur in the lens as well (lenticular astigmatism). This can be compared to the curves of a football versus a basketball. A basketball has the same curvature all the way around. A football, like astigmatism, has one curvature that is steeper than the other (the curve that you can put your hand around to pick up the ball is the steepest curvature).

Corneal astigmatism is easily measured with instruments such as a keratometer. Lenticular astigmatism is usually determined by subtracting the corneal astigmatism from the amount of cylindrical correction the patient requires for best visual acuity (refractive astigmatism). For example, if the refractive astigmatism measures 3.00 diopters at 90 degrees and the corneal astigmatism is 2.25 diopters at the same axis, there is 0.75 diopters of lenticular astigmatism at 90 degrees. While lenticular astigmatism is often added to the amount of corneal astigmatism, it is possible for it to decrease the amount of overall astigmatism. If the axis of the lenticular astigmatism is

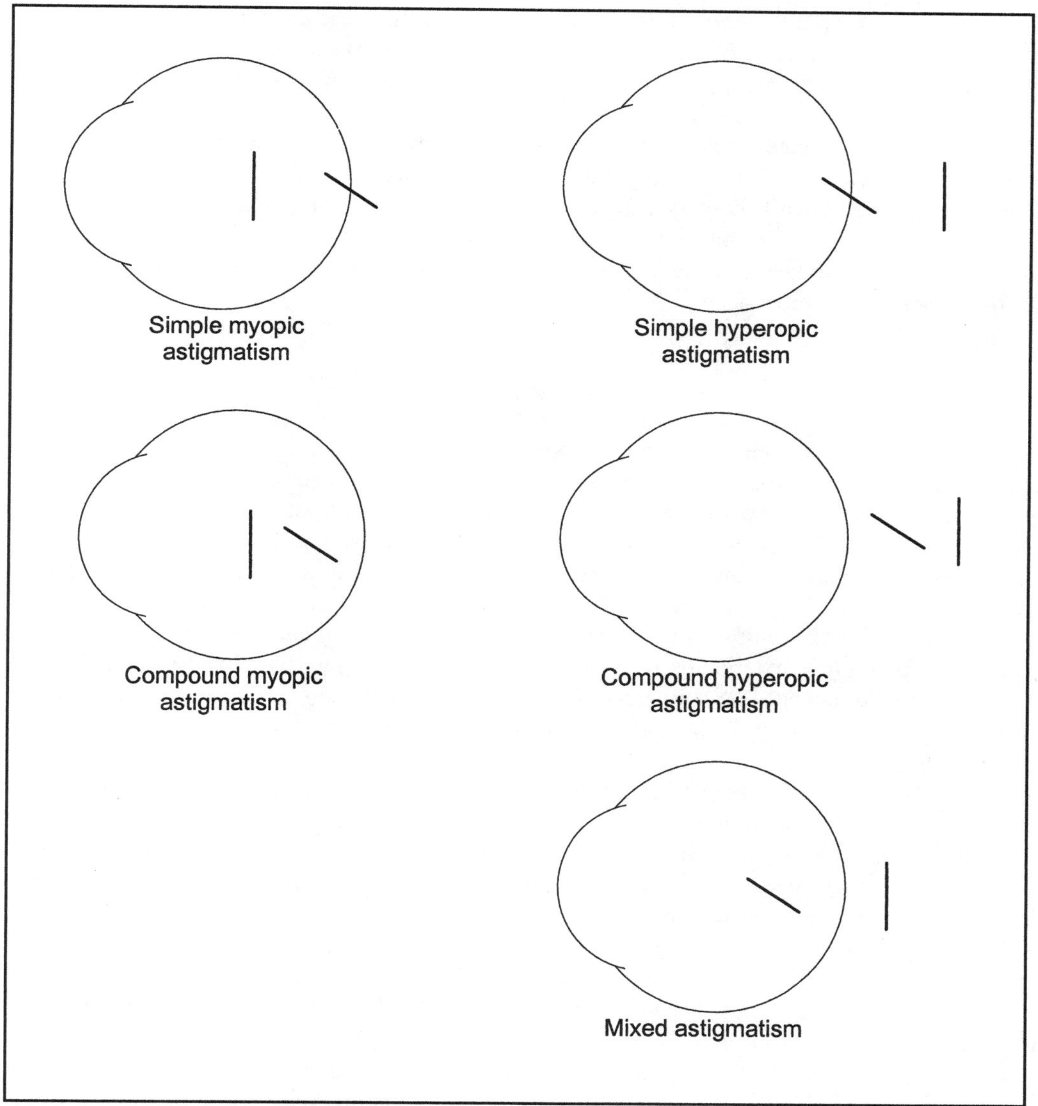

Figure 16-3. Types of astigmatism.

perpendicular to that of the corneal astigmatism, they counteract each other, causing less refractive astigmatism.

Astigmatism can be classified according to the orientation of its meridians or by where the focal lines are positioned in relation to the retina. With-the-rule astigmatism identifies the eye that has its greatest refractive power in the vertical meridian. Conversely, *against-the-rule astigmatism* is the term used to describe the eye with its maximum refractive power in the horizontal meridian. An eye with the principal meridians located more than 30 degrees away from 90 degrees or 180 degrees has oblique astigmatism.

The types of astigmatism associated with the position of the focal lines are called simple, compound, and mixed astigmatism (Figure 16-3). Simple astigmatism is present when one focal line is on the retina; in simple myopic astigmatism the second focal line is in front of the retina and in simple hyperopic astigmatism, the second focal line is "behind" the retina. Compound astigmatism has both focal lines on the same side of the retina; compound myopic astigmatism has both focal lines in front of the retina, and compound hyperopic astigmatism has both focal lines "behind" the retina. Mixed astigmatism is present when one focal line is in front of the retina and the other is behind the retina.

Eyes with uncorrected astigmatism are unable to achieve a sharp focus regardless of the distance of the object, since there are two focus lines rather than a single focus point. Small amounts of astigmatism (less than 1 diopter) tend not to cause symptoms. A larger amount of astigmatism, if left uncorrected, is often the cause of headaches along the eyebrow. (The ciliary muscle is overworked as it searches for a clear focus. The ciliary muscle does not have any pain receptors itself but can cause a brow ache.)

Presbyopia

Presbyopia is often confused with hyperopia. This is probably because the layman's term for hyperopia is farsightedness. Since nearsightedness means you can see near but not far, then the average person assumes farsightedness means one can see far, but not near. While it is true that presbyopia causes difficulties seeing near objects, it is not the same as hyperopia.

Presbyopia is derived from the Greek words *presbus* (old man) and *ops* (eye). Presbyopia is caused by a decrease in the elasticity of the crystalline lens. If we consider the embryology of the human eye, the lens develops on the outside of the eye and is then encapsulated inside the eye. Because of its origin as external tissue, it continues to grow throughout life like hair or nails, only slower. Since the old cells cannot be cut away and are not sloughed off, the cells become more compacted. The lens of an infant's eye is very pliable, but with each passing year, it becomes more rigid.

When the ciliary muscle contracts, it releases tension on the zonules that are attached to the capsule of the lens. In a young eye, this allows the lens to assume a more round (and powerful) shape. In an older eye, the lens has lost its ability to change shape, reducing the capacity to accommodate. It is also speculated that the ciliary muscle loses some of its tone with age, rendering it less able to effect the accommodative response.

The ability of the eye to change its focus naturally diminishes each year. Its effects are not usually noticed, however, until around age 40 or 45. By then, enough accommodation has been lost to make near work blurry. The early presbyope tends to move reading material further away to increase sharpness, but eventually the arm is not long enough.

Presbyopia is corrected using plus-powered spheres placed over whatever correction is required for clear distance vision. An emmetropic eye will require assistance in the way of reading glasses; the distance visual acuity remains unchanged. The hyperopic eye tends to need reading glasses earlier in life; it eventually will not be able to focus through the farsightedness and will need corrective lenses to see clearly in the distance, too. An uncorrected myopic eye is able to see clearly at its farpoint; mild myopes can read by simply removing the corrective lenses they use for seeing in the distance.

Aphakia

Aphakia is the absence of the crystalline lens, usually after it is removed because of a cataract. When cataract surgery was first developed, and for many years following, aphakia was a common finding. In the past few decades, the use of intraocular lens (IOL) implants (pseudophakia) has become the norm following cataract extraction. With each passing year, there is less likelihood of encountering someone with an aphakic eye due to cataract surgery. Alternately, the lens may be dislocated due to trauma or disease.

High hyperopia is usually seen in aphakia since the average crystalline lens accounts for +15.0 diopters of refractive power in the eye. In order for vision to be restored, this power must be replaced with a contact or spectacle lens. The exception to this situation is when moderate or high myopia existed prior to becoming aphakic. Of course, without a crystalline lens, there will also be an absence of accommodation. An aphake of any age will require bifocals or separate reading glasses.

Anisometropia

The word anisometropia is from the Greek words *anisos* (unequal), *metron* (measure), and *ops* (vision). The term is usually reserved to describe a difference in refractive error between the two eyes of 1 diopter or more. If the difference between the two eyes is high enough, aniseikonia may result (see next section).

While it is frequently asymptomatic, anisometropia can cause eyestrain, or worse, amblyopia (reduced "best" acuity without obvious cause). Amblyopia is more common in cases where one eye is hyperopic. The brain chooses to use the eye that requires the least accommodation to see clearly. Since both eyes accommodate equally, the more hyperopic eye never achieves the sharp image necessary for good visual development in preschool years.

Aniseikonia

Aniseikonia originates from the Greek words *aniso* (unequal) and *eikon* (image). It is a condition in which the size and shape of the image in one eye differs from that in the other eye. The brain may be unable to fuse the two images, resulting in an extra ghost image or diplopia. Aniseikonia is often the result of a significant amount of anisometropia, especially when corrected by spectacle lenses instead of contact lenses. Knapp's rule indicates that if the anisometropia is caused solely by a difference in the axial length (AL) of the eyes, no aniseikonia will occur if the lenses are placed 15 mm from the eye, regardless of the difference in refractive errors. However, it is quite rare for Knapp's rule to apply since there is almost always a difference in optical powers, as well as AL disparity.

The most common situation in which aniseikonia exists occurs as a result of surgery. For example, for a patient who has a significant refractive error and undergoes cataract (or refractive) surgery on one eye, the refractive error is minimized in the surgical eye, but the other eye still requires a strong corrective lens for clear vision. Other times, both eyes may have had cataract surgery, but the wrong IOL power was used in one eye (or both).

Antimetropia

The origin of the word antimetropia comes from the Greek words *anti* (against), *metron* (measure), and *ops* (vision). It is a condition in which one eye is myopic and the other is hyperopic. In mild cases, antimetropia is usually well tolerated. The hyperopic eye is used primarily for distance vision while the myopic eye is used for reading. High degrees of antimetropia (over 4 diopters) typically cause aniseikonia.

Evaluating Refractive Errors

Refractometry is the basic method of evaluating refractive errors. (This is different from a refraction; refractometry is the measurement itself, and a refraction involves generating a lens prescription from that measurement.) This can be done using loose *"trial" lenses* and a *trial frame* or a *refractor* (also called phoropter). It is a subjective test that requires input from the patient.

Objective methods of measuring refractive errors include *retinoscopy* in which the examiner evaluates the nature of the instrument's light as reflected off the retina. The principles of analyzing light projected onto the retina are also used in computerized *autorefractors*, which give a print-out of a base-line measurement.

Any test that evaluates the refractive power of the cornea (such as *keratometry* and *corneal topography*) can also be considered at least a partial measurement of refractive error.

Refractive errors like myopia, hyperopia, and astigmatism are considered lower-order aberrations (distortions caused by imperfections in the optical system). These are correctable with glasses or contact lenses. However, there are other imperfections in the average eye that leave some aberrations that normal spectacles will not correct—these are higher-order aberrations. An *aberrometer* (or *wavefront analyzer*) can be used to detect these impurities in the optical system. In most cases, the higher-order aberrations are asymptomatic. In more severe cases, halos and/or starburst effects can occur at night, and a general blurriness may be noticed during the day. The information gleaned from aberrometry can be used to produce wavefront-corrected spectacles or contact lenses, or to allow a wavefront-guided refractive laser treatment to be performed.

Glossary of Common Disorders

amblyopia: Permanent decrease in vision caused by lack of clear vision during early childhood. Usually affects one eye but can easily be bilateral. Can be caused by conditions such as significant anisometropia, cataracts, or strabismus. If clear vision in each eye is not obtained before the brain has finished developing the ability to see, amblyopia is likely to occur.

ametropia: Presence of any refractive error, such as myopia, hyperopia, and/or astigmatism.

anisometropia: A difference in the refractive error between the two eyes; can lead to aniseikonia (a difference in the size of retinal images between the two eyes) if there is more than 3 diopters difference between the two eyes.

astigmatism: Refractive error that is not equal in all meridians. Most common is regular astigmatism in which the axis of the least amount of focus is perpendicular to the axis of the highest amount of focus and is easily corrected with cylindrical lenses. Irregular astigmatism can occur as a result of injuries or ocular disorders that create an uneven refractive surface.

emmetropia: No refractive error is present. Distant objects focus on the retina when no accommodation is exerted.

hyperopia (farsightedness): Refractive error that occurs when there is insufficient focusing power to bring light to a focus on the retina. Can be absolute where there is not enough accommodation to create the extra focus required, or latent where the accommodative ability of the eye can meet the focusing needs of the eye, or a combination of absolute and latent (total hyperopia). Plus-powered, or convex, lenses are used to correct hyperopia.

malignant myopia: Progressive myopia that is associated with a thinning of the sclera and retina.

myopia (nearsightedness): Refractive error that has near objects in focus, but distant objects are blurred. Occurs when the focusing power of the eye's cornea and crystalline lens (without accommodation) exceeds the amount needed for the length of the eye. Minus-powered, or concave, lenses are used to correct myopia.

presbyopia: Decreased accommodation that manifests when there is insufficient accommodation present to bring near objects into focus.

Bibliography

Abelson MB, Alfonso E. *Papillary Update: Mydriasis and Miosis During Surgery.* Princeton, NJ: Excerpta Medica; 1986.

Adler FR. *Textbook of Ophthalmology.* 7th ed. Philadelphia, PA: WB Saunders Company; 1962.

Asrani S, Zeimer R, Goldberg MF, Zou, S. Serial optical sectioning of macular holes at different stages of development. *Ophthalmology*. 1999;106:1145-1151.

Bagga H, Greenfield DS, Feuer W, Knighton RW. Scanning laser polimetry with variable cornea compensation and optical coherence tomography in normal and glaucomatous eyes. *Am J Ophthalmol.* 2003;135:521-529.

Berliner ML. *Biomicroscopy of the Eye: Slit Lamp Microscopy of the Living Eye.* Vol 1. New York, NY: Paul B. Hoeber Incorporated (Medical Book Department of Harper & Brothers); 1949.

Brooks CW, Borish IM. *System for Ophthalmic Dispensing*. 2nd ed. Newton, MA: Butterworth-Heinemann; 1996.

Camara JE, Bengzon AU. Nasolacrimal Duct, Obstruction. eMedicine from WebMD. http://www.emedicine.com/oph/topic465.htm Accessed August 3, 2006.

Cassin B. *Fundamentals for Ophthalmic Medical Personnel.* Philadelphia, PA: WB Saunders Company; 1995.

Chumbley LC. *Ophthalmology in Internal Medicine.* Philadelphia, PA: WB Saunders Company; 1981.

Cook CS, Ozanics V, Jakobiec FA. Prenatal development of the eye and its adnexa. In: Tasman W, Jeager EA, eds. *Duane's Ophthalmology on CD-ROM.* Philadelphia, PA: Lippincott-Raven Publishers; 1996.

Cordes FC. *Cataract Types.* Rochester, MN: American Academy of Ophthalmology and Otolaryngology; 1961.

de Grouchy J, Turleau C. *Clinical Atlas of Human Chromosomes.* New York, NY: John Wiley and Sons; 1977.

Diamond Group. *The Brain: A User's Manual.* New York, NY: Berkley Publishing Corporation; 1983.

Diamond S, Medina J. *Headaches: Clinical Symposia.* Vol 33, No 2. Summit, NJ: CIBA Pharmaceuticals Company; 1981.

Donaldson D. Cornea and sclera. In: Donaldson D, ed. *Atlas of External Diseases of the Eye.* 2nd ed. St. Louis, MO: C.V. Mosby Company; 1980.

Drexler W, Morgner U, Ghanta RK, Kartner FX, Schuman JS, Fujimoto JG. Ultrahigh-resolution ophthalmic optical coherence tomography. *Nat Med.* 2001;7:502-507.

Duane TD, ed. *Biomedical Foundations of Ophthalmology.* Vol 1-3. New York, NY: Harper & Row; 1982.

Duane TD, ed. *Clinical Ophthalmology*. Vol 1-5. Philadelphia, PA: Harper & Rowe; 1983.

Duane TD, ed. *Clinical Ophthalmology.* Vol 1-5. Philadelphia, PA: J.B. Lippincott; 1987.

Duane TD, Jaeger EA. *Biomedical Foundations of Ophthalmology.* Philadelphia, PA: JB Lippincott; 1991.

Duane TD, Jaeger EA. *Biomedical Foundations of Ophthalmology.* Philadelphia, PA: JB Lippincott: 1996.

Duke-Elder S. *System of Ophthalmology*. Vols 2, 8, and 13. London: Kimpton Publishers; 1961.

External Disease and Cornea. Section 7: Basic and clinical science course. San Francisco, CA: American Academy of Ophthalmology; 1985.

Fedor P, Kaufman SC. Corneal Topography and Imaging. eMedicine from WebMD. http://www.emedicine.com/oph/topic711.htm Accessed August 12, 2006.

Fraunfelder F, Roy FH. *Current Ocular Therapy.* Philadelphia, PA: WB Saunders Company; 1980.

Fundamentals and Principles of Ophthalmology. Section 1: Basic and Clinical Science Course. San Francisco, CA: American Academy of Ophthalmology; 1988-1989.

Gayton JL, Ledford JR. *The Crystal Clear Guide to Sight for Life.* Lancaster, PA: Starburst Publishers; 1996.

General Medical Case Problems. Section 10: Basic and clinical science course. Rochester, MN: American Academy of Ophthalmology and Otolaryngology; 1977.

Gittinger JW. *Ophthalmology: A Clinical Introduction.* Boston, MA: Little, Brown and Company; 1980.

Grayson M. *Diseases of the Cornea.* St. Louis, MO: C.V. Mosby Company; 1979.

Grosvenor T. *Primary Care Optometry.* 3rd ed. Newton, MA: Butterworth-Heinemann; 1996.

Hansen VC. *Ocular Motility.* Thorofare, NJ: SLACK Incorporated; 1990.

Huang D, Kaiser PK, Lowder CY, Traboulsi EI. *Retinal Imaging.* Philadelphia PA: Elsevier; 2006.

Havener WH. *Synopsis of Ophthalmology.* 5th ed. St. Louis, MO: C.V. Mosby Company; 1979.

Heart Facts. Dallas, Tex: American Heart Association; 1980.

Jones DB, Liesegang TJ, Robinson NM. *Laboratory Diagnosis of Ocular Infections.* Washington, DC: American Society for Microbiology; 1981.

Jones LT, Reich MJ, Wirtschafter JD. *Ophthalmic Anatomy.* Rochester, MN: American Academy of Ophthalmology and Otolaryngology; 1971.

Kagemann L, Harris A, Jonescu-Cuypers C, et al. Comparison of ocular hemodynamics measured by a new retinal blood flowmeter and color Doppler imaging. *Ophthalmic Surg Lasers Imaging.* 2003;87:622-625.

Kapit W, Elson LM. *The Anatomy Coloring Book.* New York, NY: Harper & Row; 1977.

Karesh JW. Topographic anatomy of the eye: an overview. In: Tasman W, Jeager EA, eds. *Duane's Ophthalmology on CD-ROM.* Philadelphia, PA: Lippincott-Raven Publishers; 1996.

Kiryu J, Shahidi M, Ogura Y, Blair NP, Zeimer R. Illustration of the stages of idiopathic macular holes by laser biomicroscopy. *Arch Ophthalmol.* 1995;113:1156-1160.

Ledford JK, Hoffman J. *Quick Reference Dictionary of Eyecare Terminology.* 5th ed. Thorofare, NJ: SLACK Incorporated; 2008.

Ledford JK, Sanders VN. *The Slit Lamp Primer.* 2nd ed. Thorofare, NJ: SLACK Incorporated; 2006.

MacDonald IM. Genetics for Ophthalmologists. Review of Ophthalmology online. http://www.revophth.com/1999/july_articles/799%20genetics.htm Accessed August 12, 2006.

Marieb EN. *Human Anatomy and Physiology.* Redwood City, CA: Benjamin/Cummings Publishing Company, Inc; 1989.

Maysolf FA. *The Eye and Systemic Disease.* St. Louis, MO: C.V. Mosby Company; 1975.

McKusick VA. *Mendelian Inheritance in Man.* 8th ed. Baltimore, MD: John Hopkins University Press; 1988.

Moses RA. *Adler's Physiology of the Eye: Clinical Applications.* 5th ed. St. Louis, MO: C.V. Mosby Company; 1970.

Moses RA. *Adler's Physiology of the Eye, Clinical Application.* 6th ed. St. Louis, MO: C.V. Mosby Company; 1975.

Muench KH. *Genetic Medicine.* New York, NY: Elsevier; 1988.

Mulvihill ML. *Human Diseases, A Systemic Approach.* 4th ed. Norwalk, CT: Appleton & Lange; 1995.

Nemeth, SC, Shea, CA. *Medical Sciences for the Ophthalmic Assistant.* Thorofare, NJ: SLACK Incorporated; 1988.

Orbit, Eyelids, and Lacrimal System. Section 9, Basic and clinical science course. San Francisco, CA: American Academy of Ophthalmology; 1985.

Pavan-Langston D. *Manual of Ocular Diagnosis and Therapy.* Boston, MA: Little, Brown and Company; 1980.

Peyman GA, Sanders DR, Goldberg MF, eds. *Principles and Practice of Ophthalmology.* Vol 1. Philadelphia, PA: WB Saunders Company; 1980.

Pou Carlos R. *Lacrimal Drainage System. Ophthalmic Hyperguide™.* www.ophthalmic.hyperguides.com Accessed August 2, 2006.

Raven PH, Johnson GB. *Biology.* 3rd ed. Dubuque, IA: Wm. C. Brown Publishers; 1995.

Renie WA, ed. *Goldberg's Genetic and Metabolic Eye Diseases*. 2nd ed. Boston, MA: Little, Brown and Company; 1986.

Scheie HG, Albert DM. *Textbook of Ophthalmology*. Philadelphia, PA: WB Saunders Company; 1977.

Sigelman J. *Retinal Diseases: Pathogenesis, Laser Therapy, and Surgery.* Boston, MA: Little, Brown and Company; 1984.

Singh D, Singh JR, Kumar V. Prenatal diagnosis for congenital malformations and genetic disorders. http://www.emedicine.com/oph/topic485.htm. Accessed August 7, 2006.

Smolin G, Thoft RA. *The Cornea.* Boston, MA: Little, Brown and Company; 1983.

Snell RS, Lemp MA. *Clinical Anatomy of the Eye*. Cambridge, MA: Blackwell Scientific Publications; 1981.

Stanbury JB, Wyngaarden JB, Fredrickson DS. *Metabolic Basis of Inherited Diseases*. 5th ed. New York, NY: McGraw Hill; 1983.

Vaughan D, Asbury T. *General Ophthalmology.* 9th ed. Los Altos, CA: Lange Medical Publications; 1980.

Vaughan D, Asbury T, Riordan-Eva P. *General Ophthalmology.* 14th ed. Norwalk, CT: Appleton & Lange; 1995.

Warwick R. *Anatomy of the Eye and Orbit.* Philadelphia, PA: WB Saunders Company; 1976.

Watsky MA, Olsen TW, Edelhauser HF. Cornea and sclera. In: Tasman W, Jeager EA, eds. *Duane's Ophthalmology on CD-ROM.* Philadelphia, PA: Lippincott-Raven Publishers; 1996.

Weatherall DJ. *The New Genetics and Clinical Practice.* New York, NY: Oxford University Press; 1985.

Wojkowski M, Lowalczyk A, Leitgeb R, Fercher AF. Full range complex spectral optical coherence tomography technique in eye imaging. *Opt Lett.* 2002;27:1415-1417.

Wojtkowski M, Bajraszewski T, Targowski P, Kowalczyk A. Real-time in vivo imaging by high-speed spectral optical coherence tomography. *Opt Lett.* 2003;28:1745-1747.

Wojtkowski M, Leitgeb R, Kowalczyk A, Bajraszewski T, Gercher AF. In vivo retinal imaging by Fourier domain optical coherence tomography. *J Biomed Opt.* 2002;7:457-463.

Wolff E, Last RJ. *Anatomy of the Eye and Orbit.* 6th ed. Philadelphia, PA: WB Saunders Company; 1968.

Index

Note: Only common disorders that are mentioned in the text itself are listed in the index; those referenced solely in the glossary following each chapter are not included here.